Adventures In Nursing

Nursing Themed Coloring Pages to Promote Relaxation

Lindsay Pawlak-Mayall

Copyright ©2018 Lindsay Pawlak-Mayall
All rights reserved. No part of this book may be reproduced or transmitted in any form, by any means, electronic or mechanical, including photocopying, scanning and recording, or by any information storage and retrieval system, without the express written consent of the author, except for the inclusion for a product review.

Thank-you for purchasing the Adventures in Nursing Coloring Book! This book was inspired by my belief that nurses everywhere deserve self-care. Nursing is a challenging career, and nurses are so giving of themselves, that they often forget that they need care too. Coloring is a therapeutic way to unwind, relax, and recharge. Each of these images were hand drawn, to reflect an element of the nursing profession. Please enjoy!

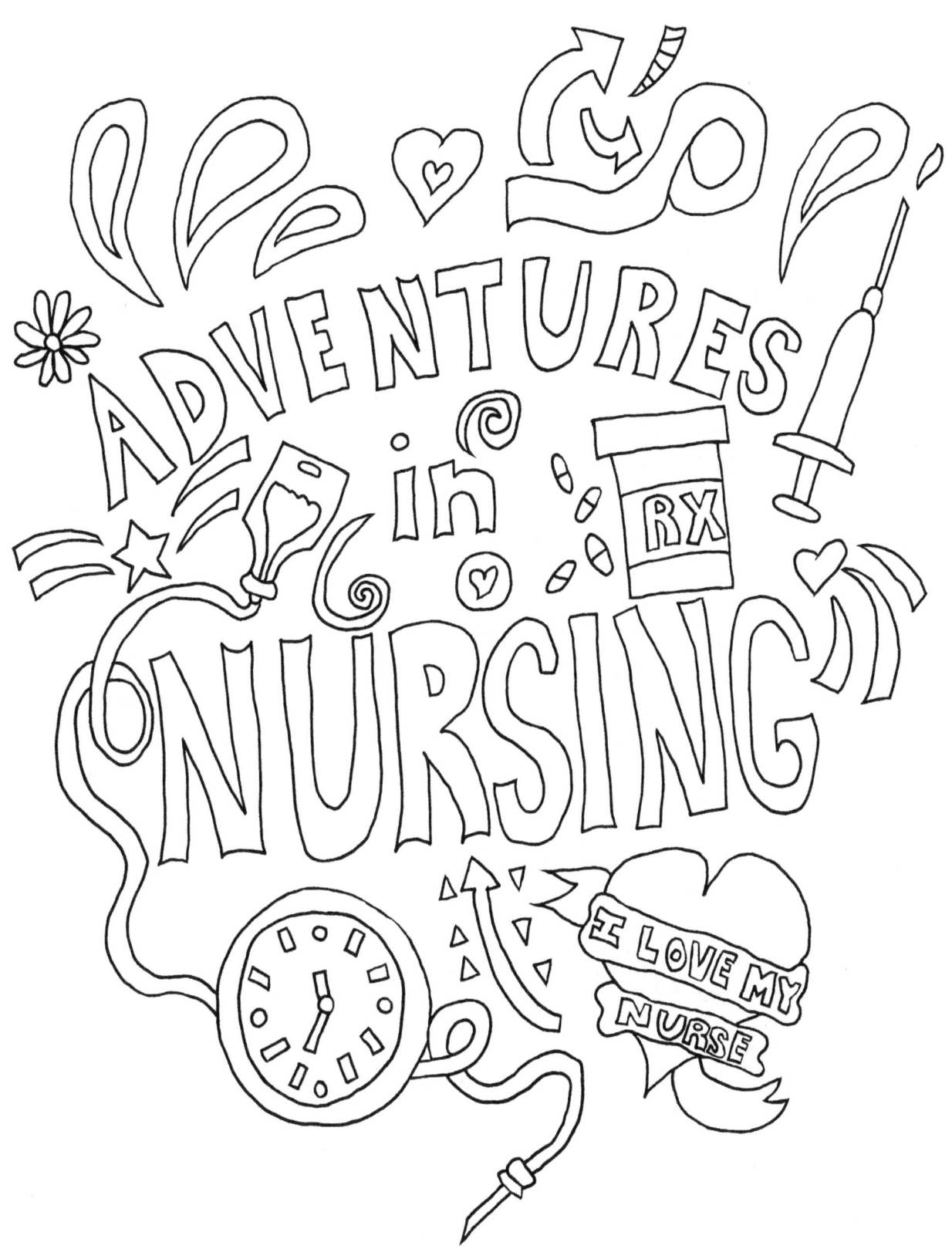

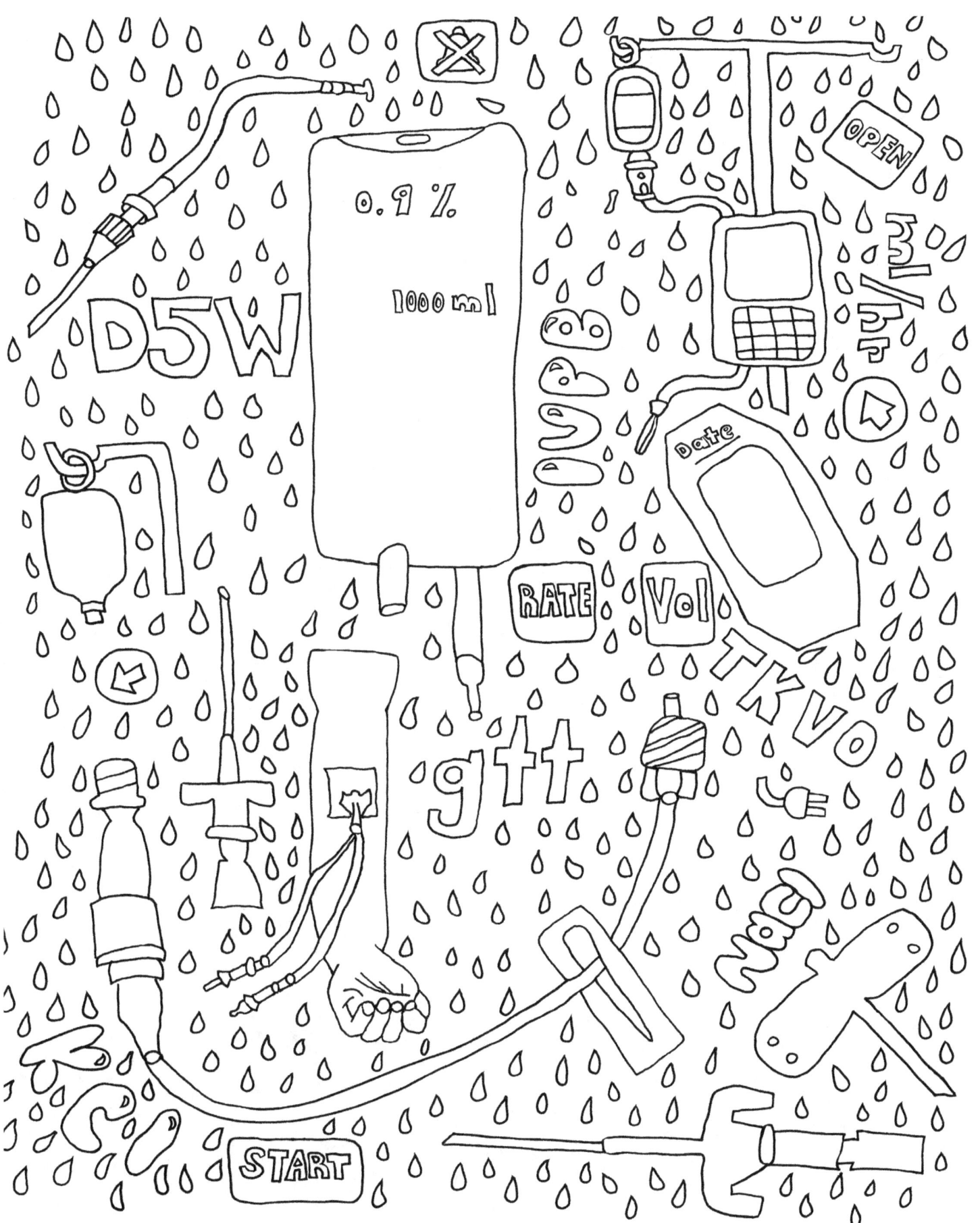

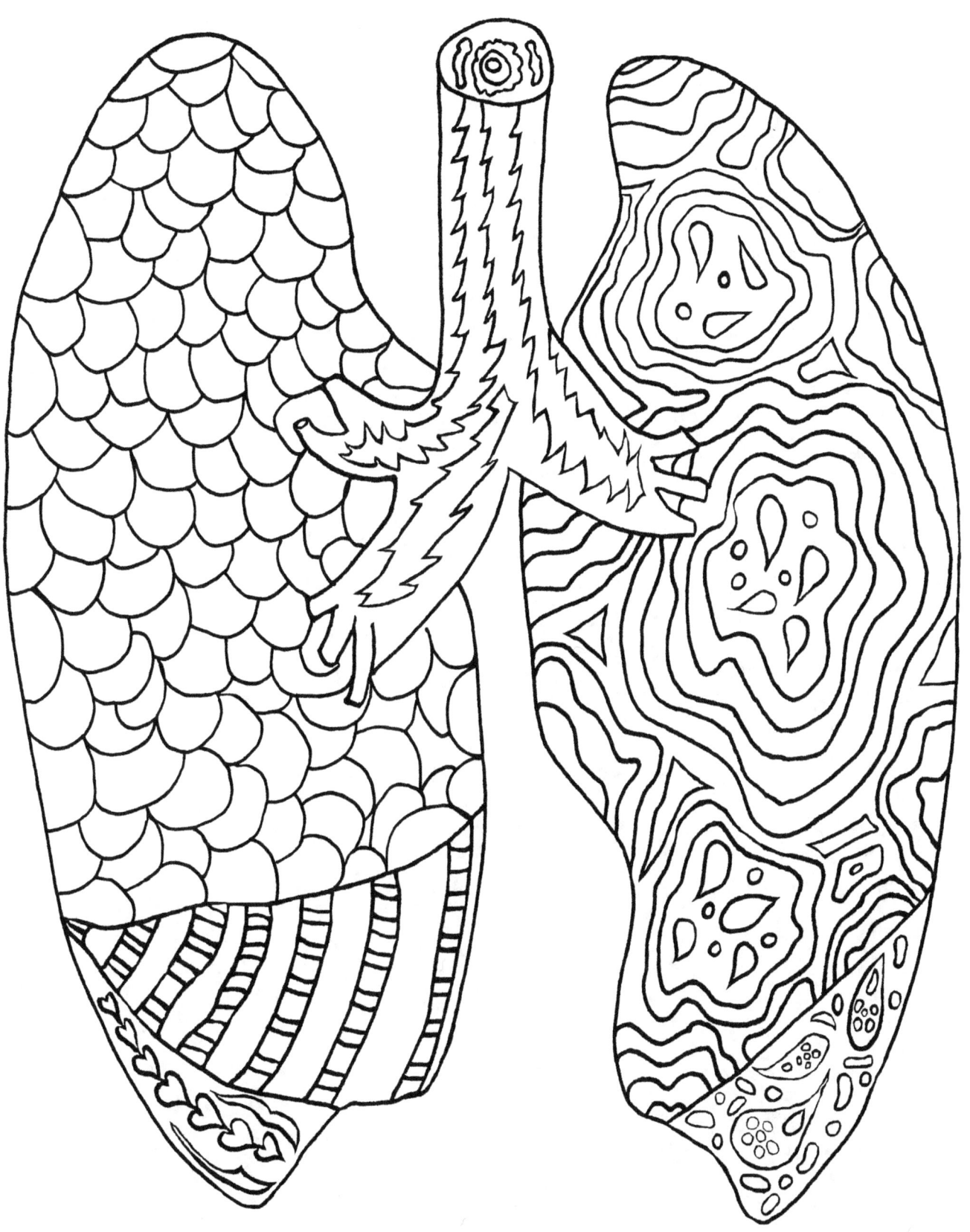

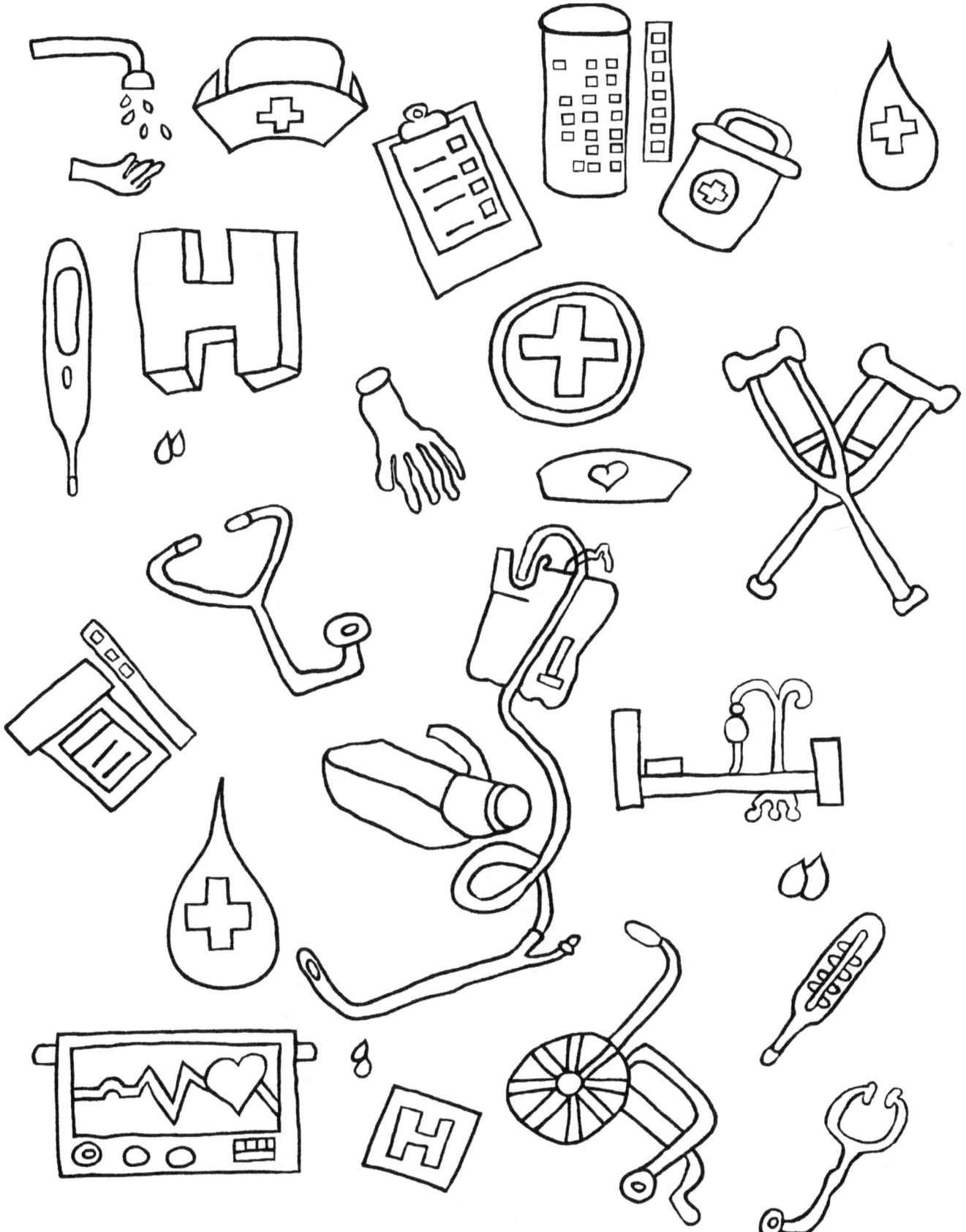

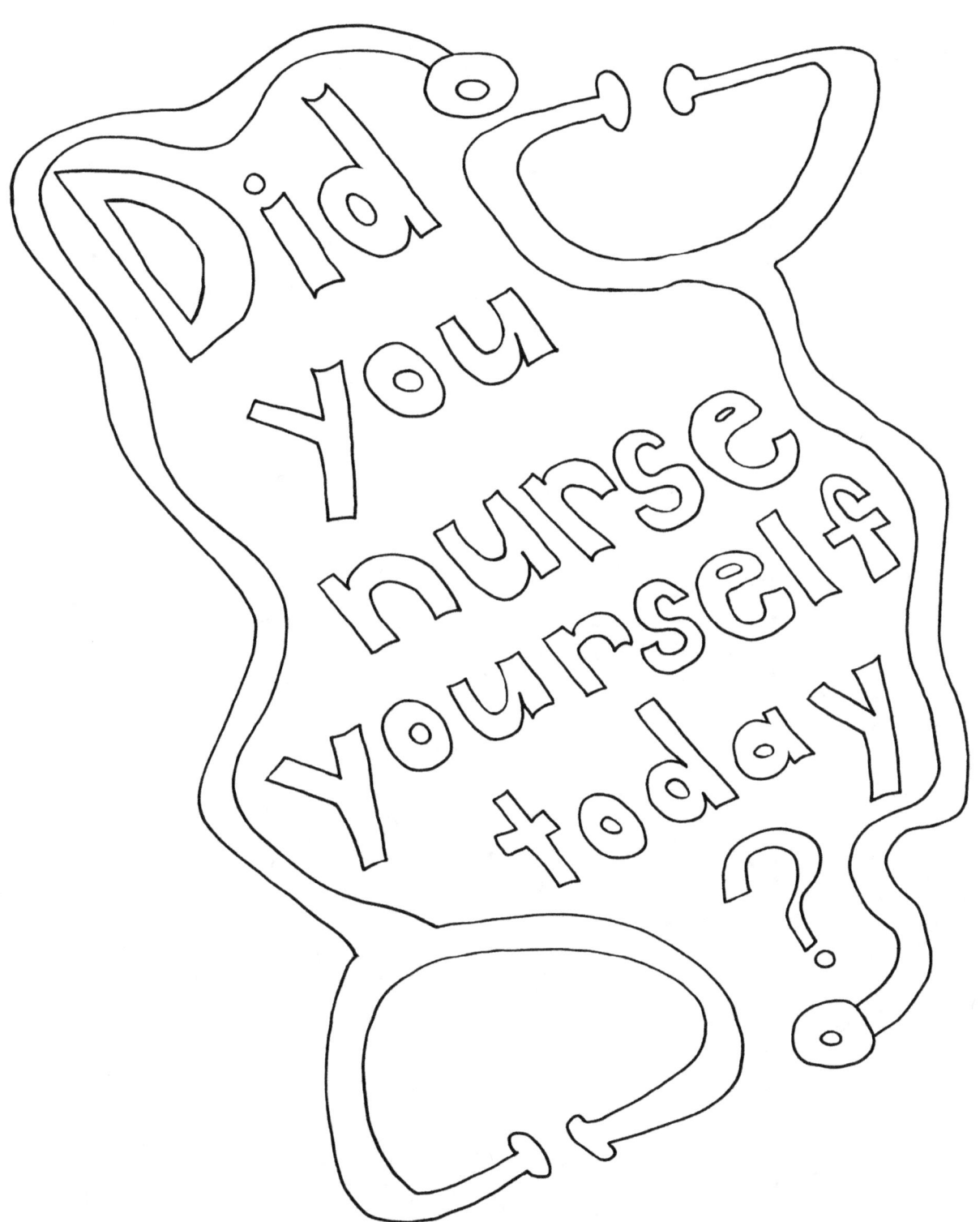

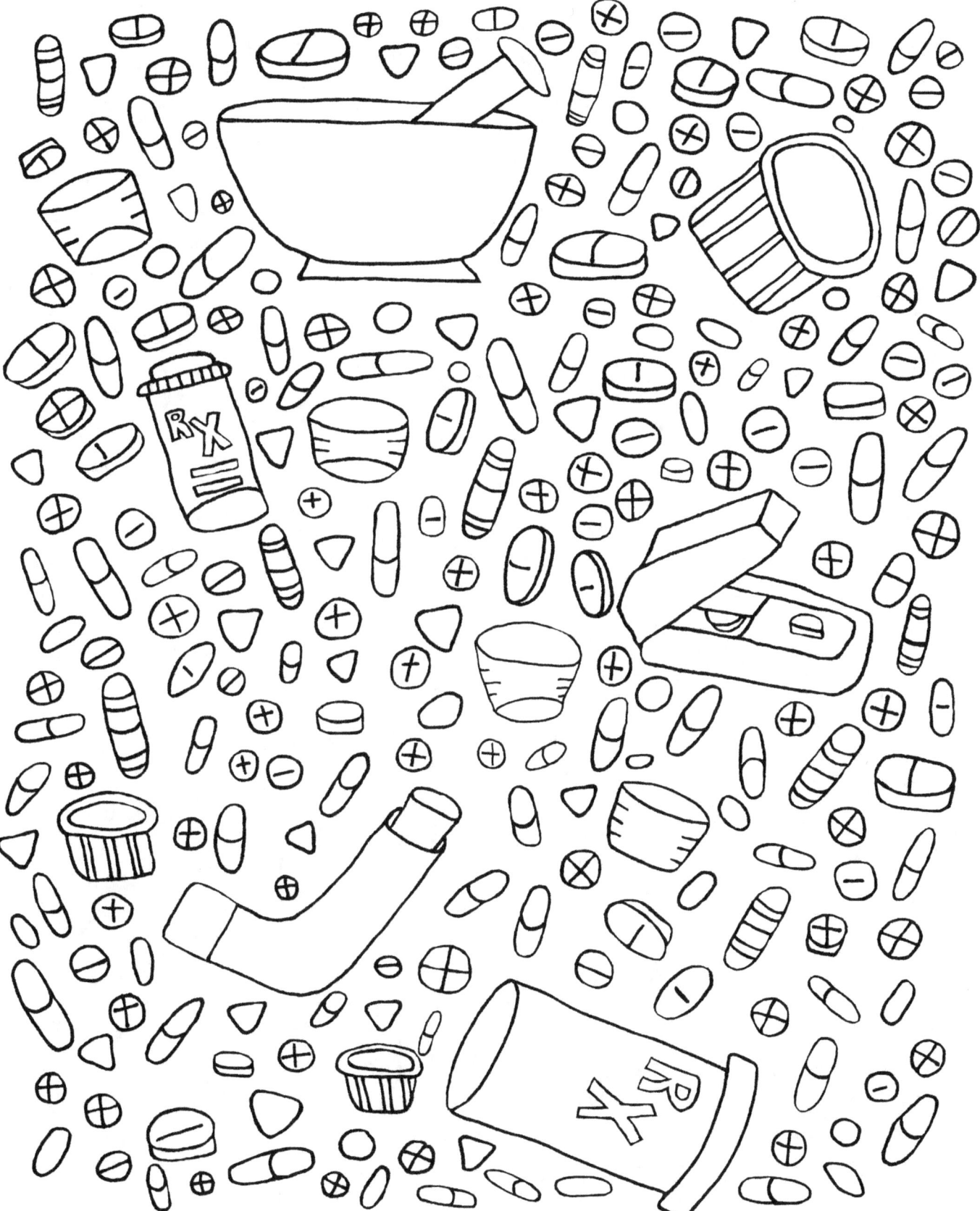

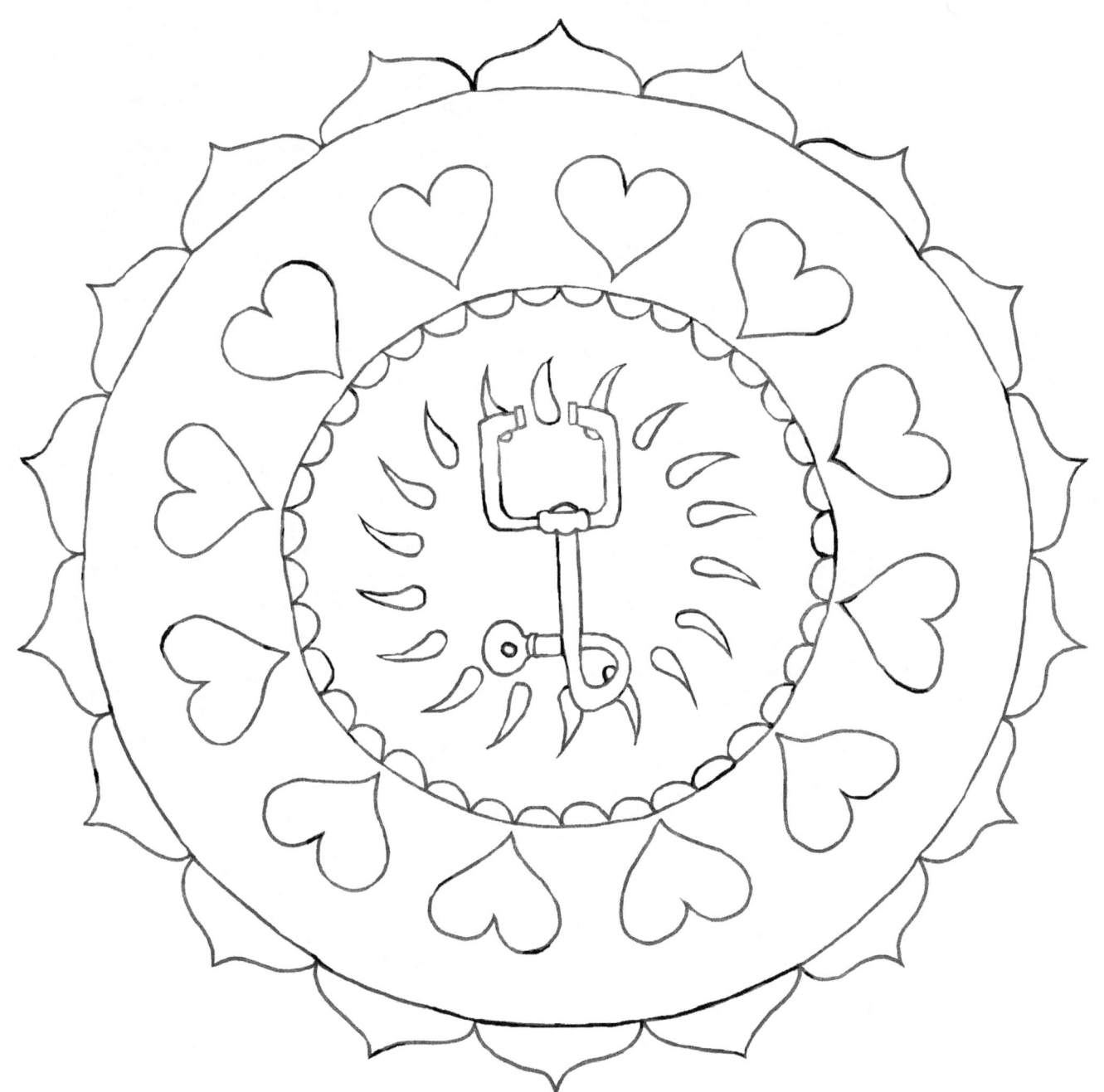

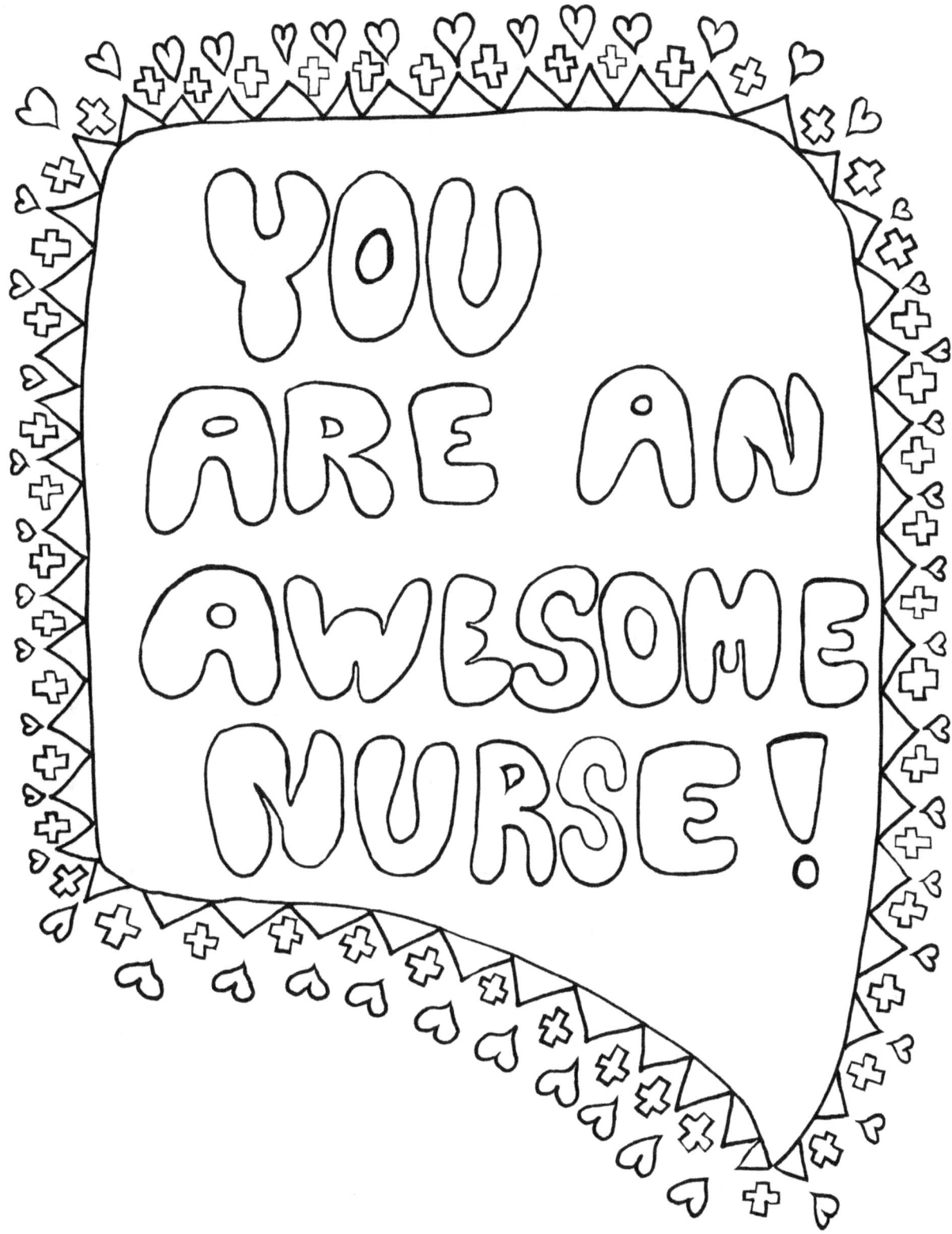

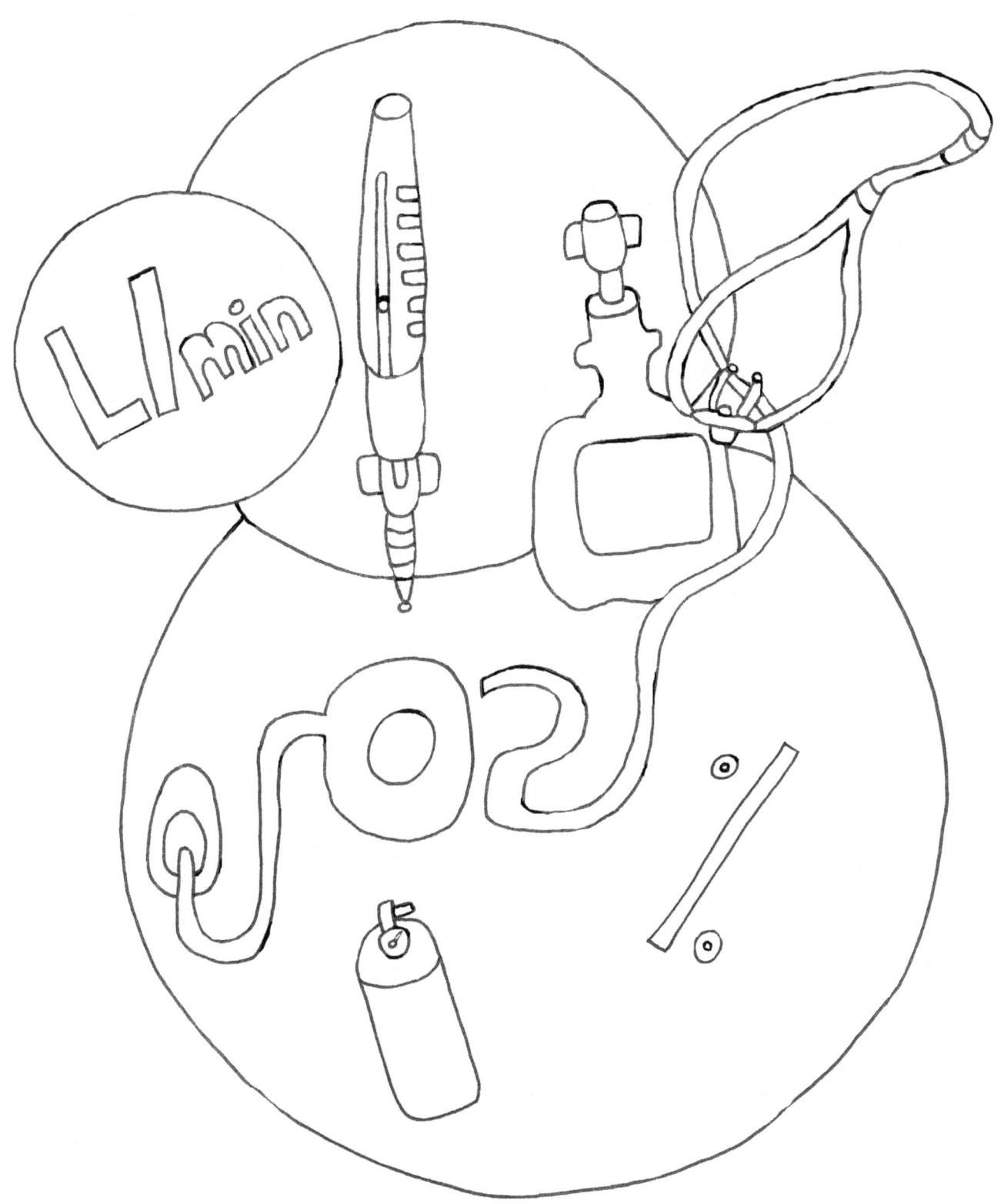

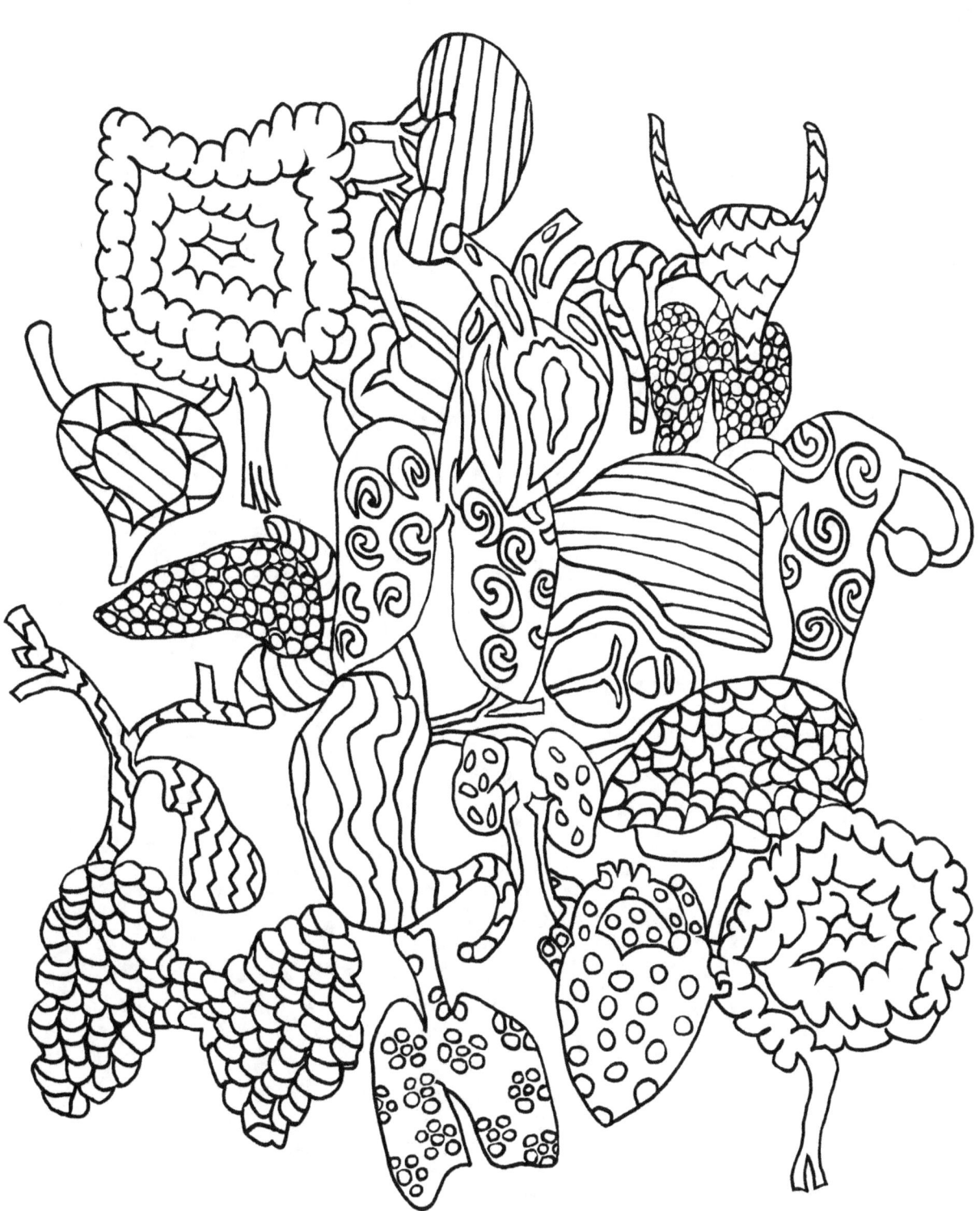

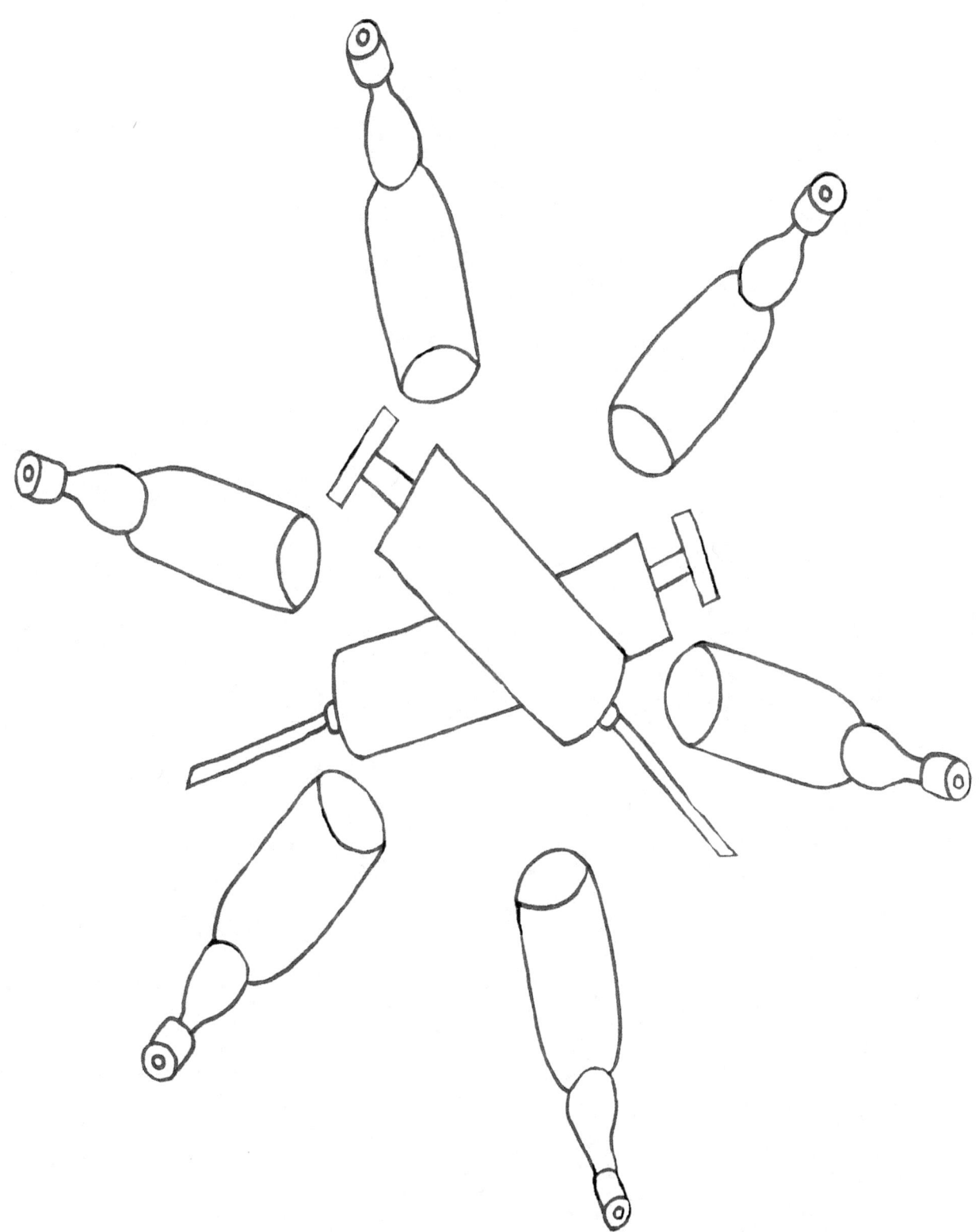

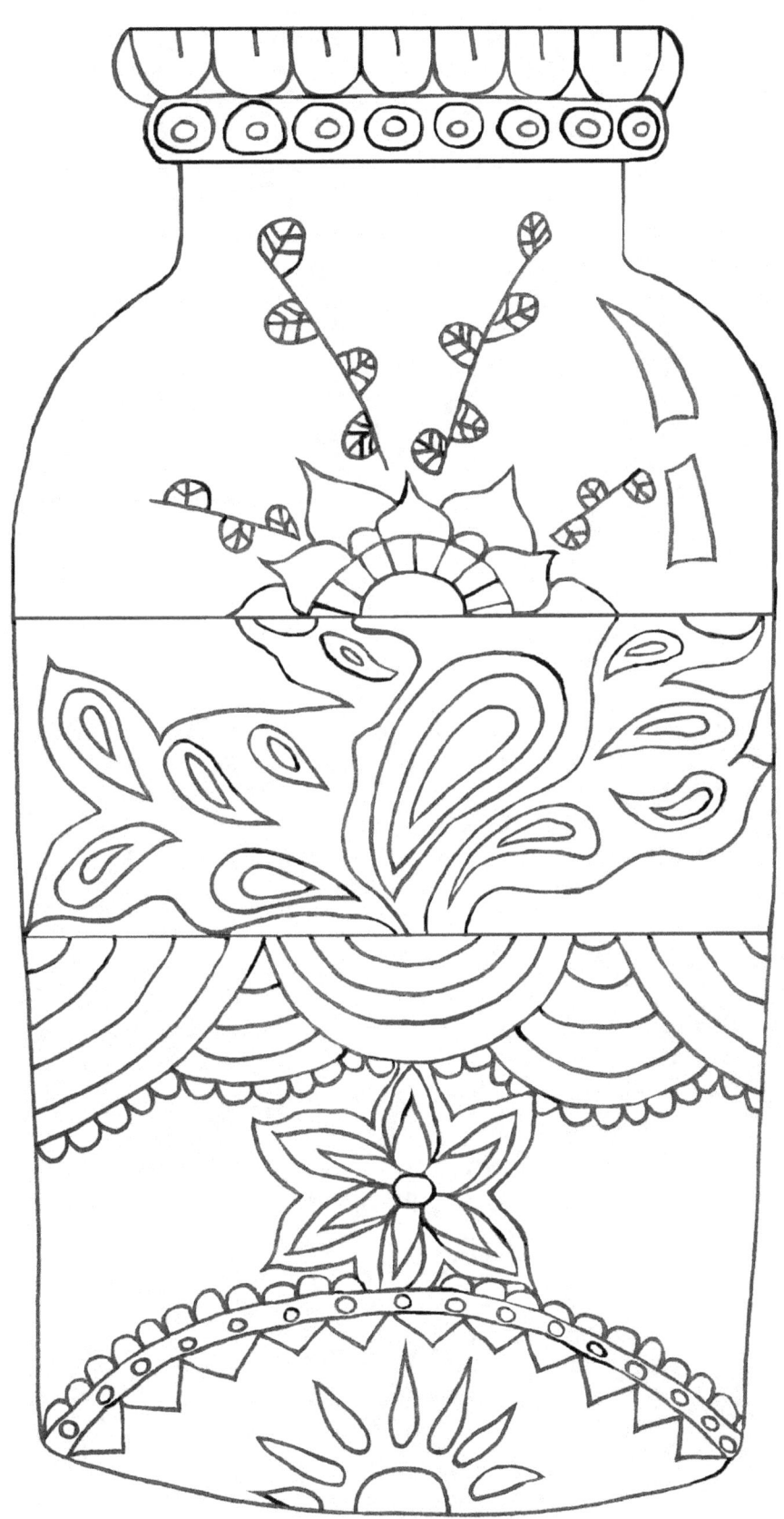

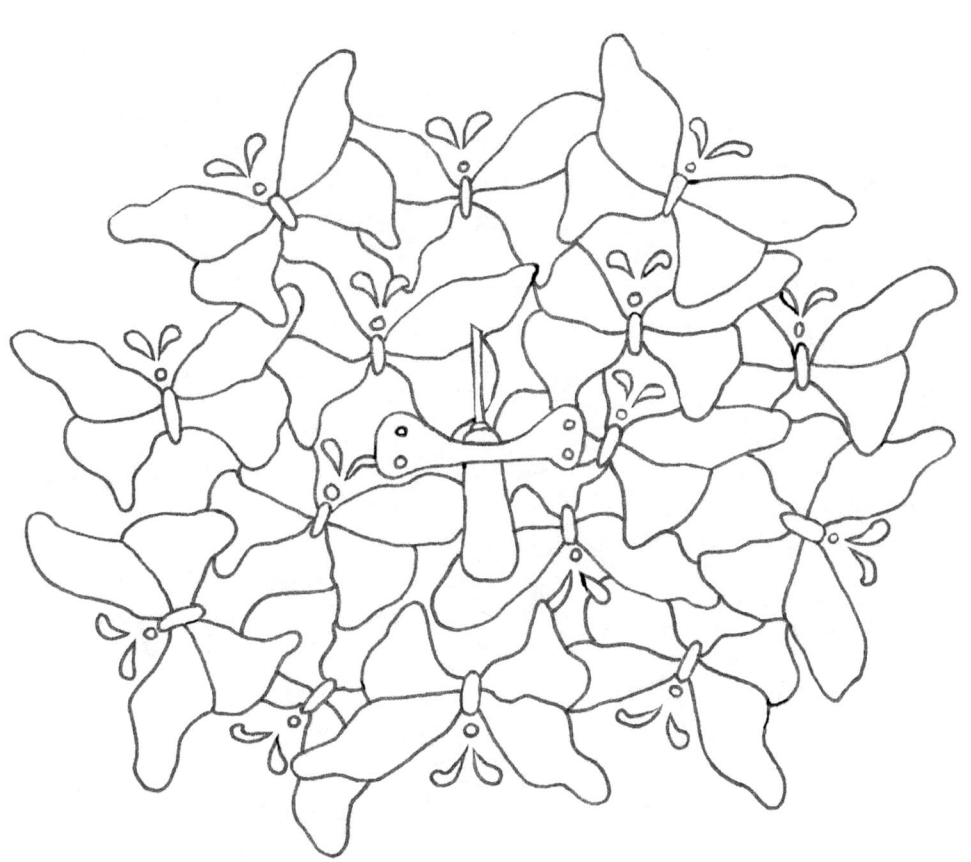

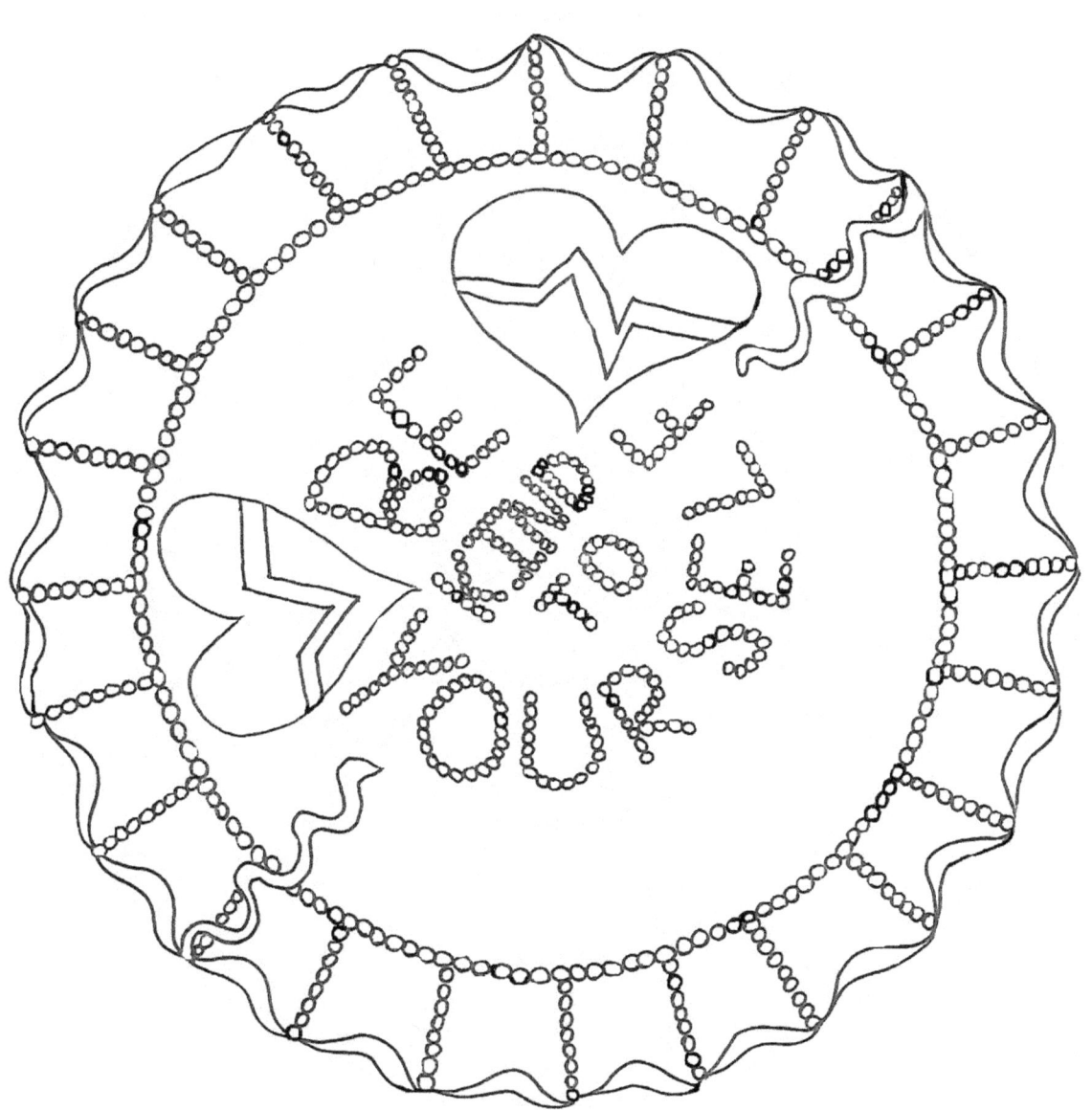

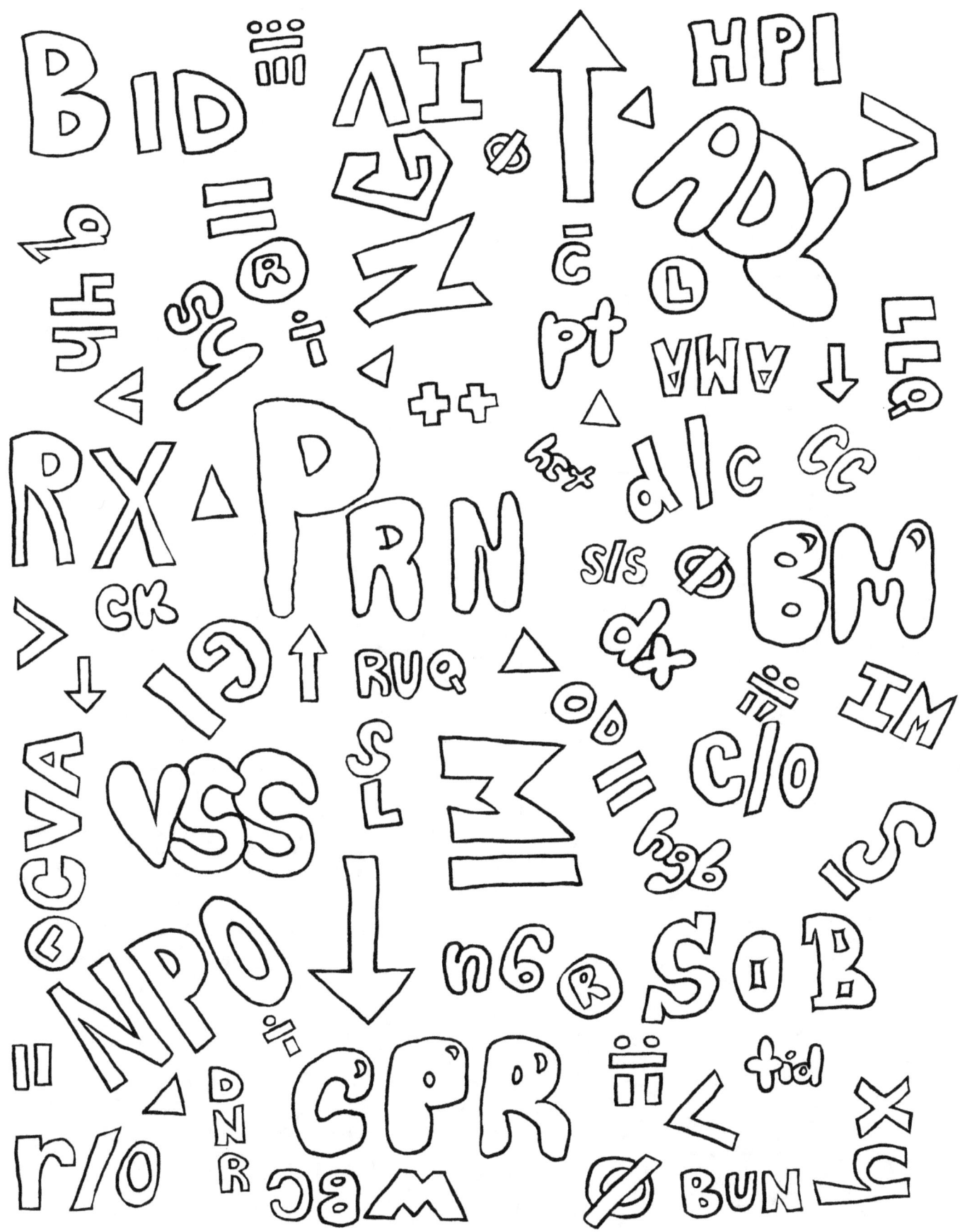

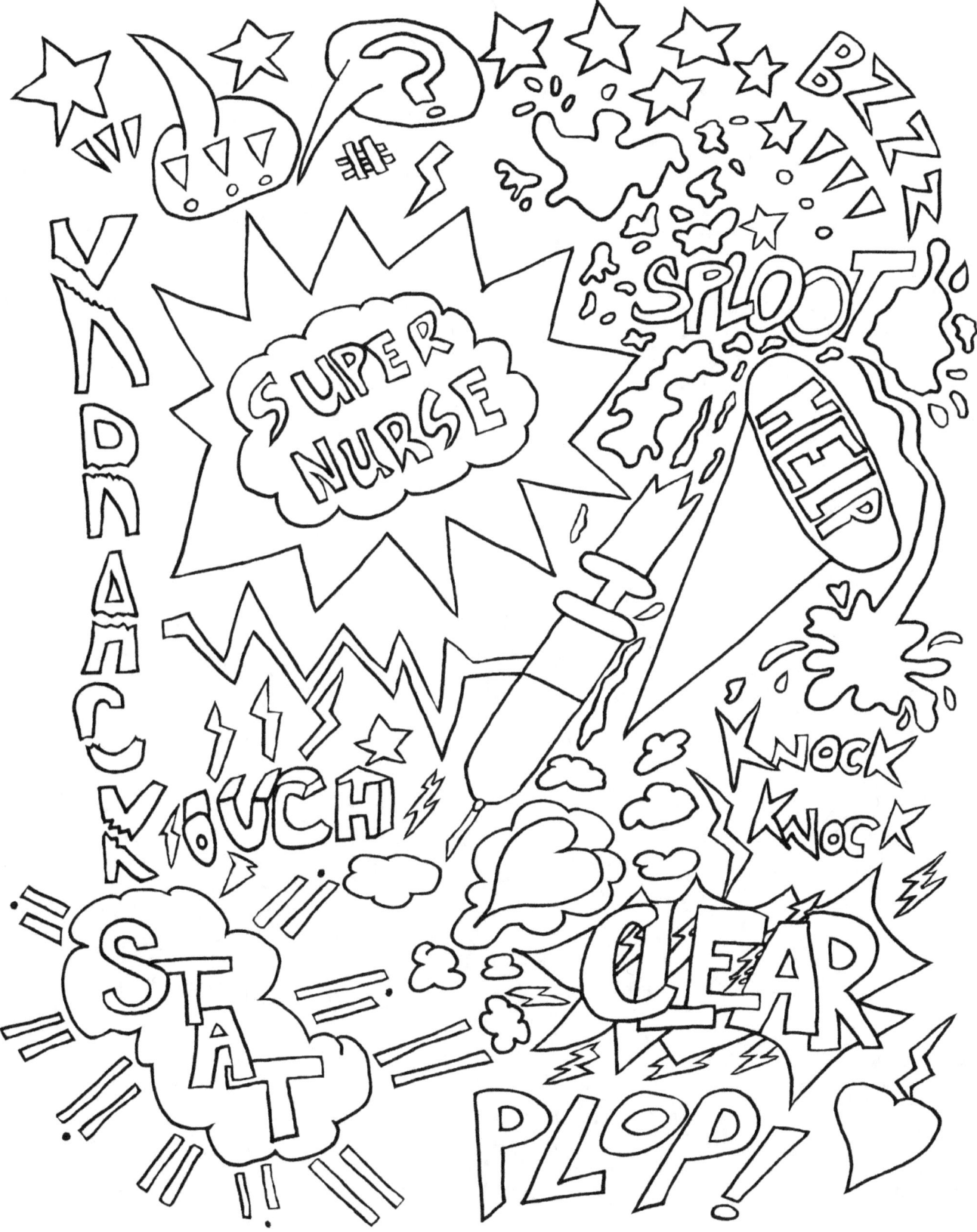

This Won't Hurt A Bit

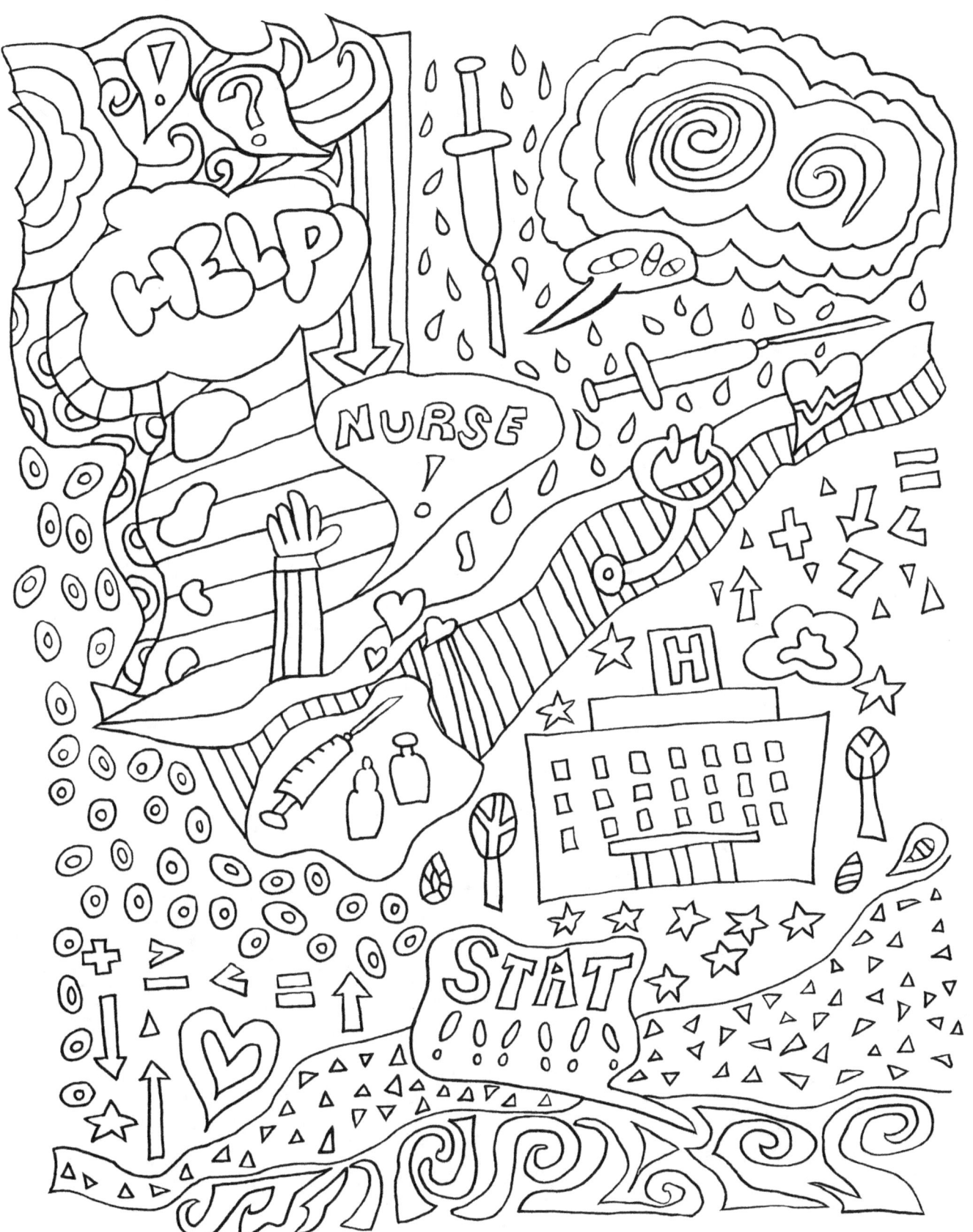

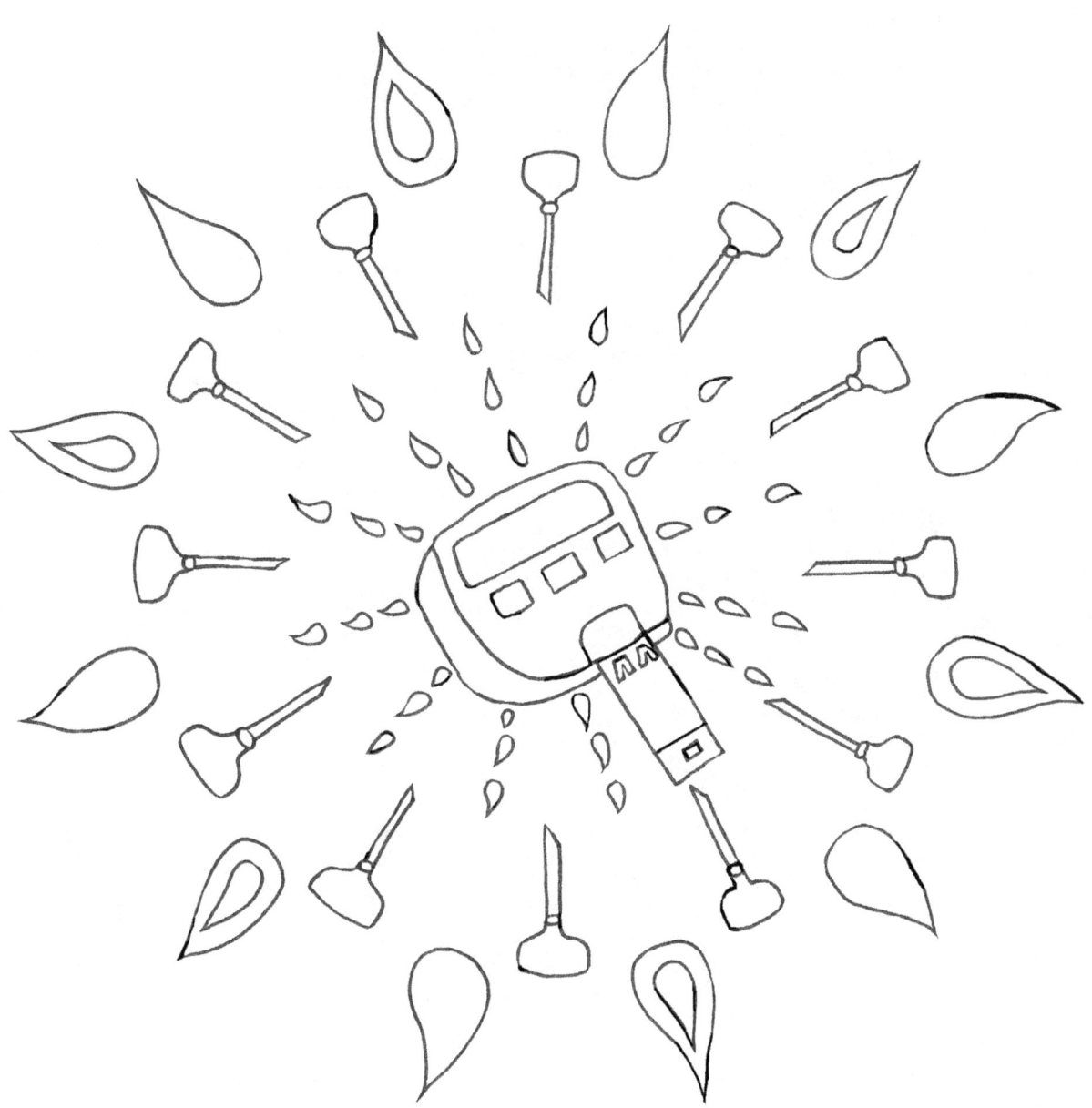

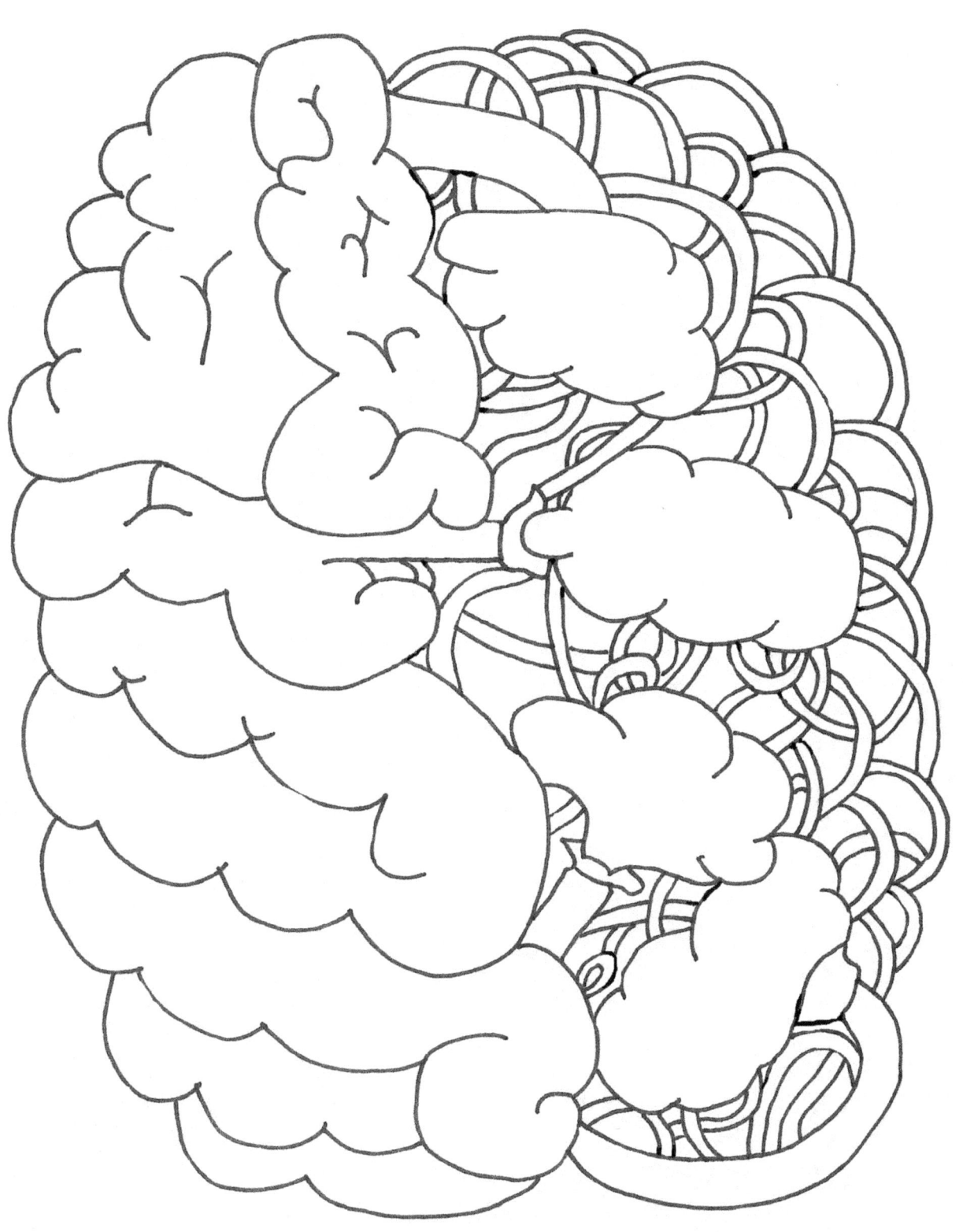

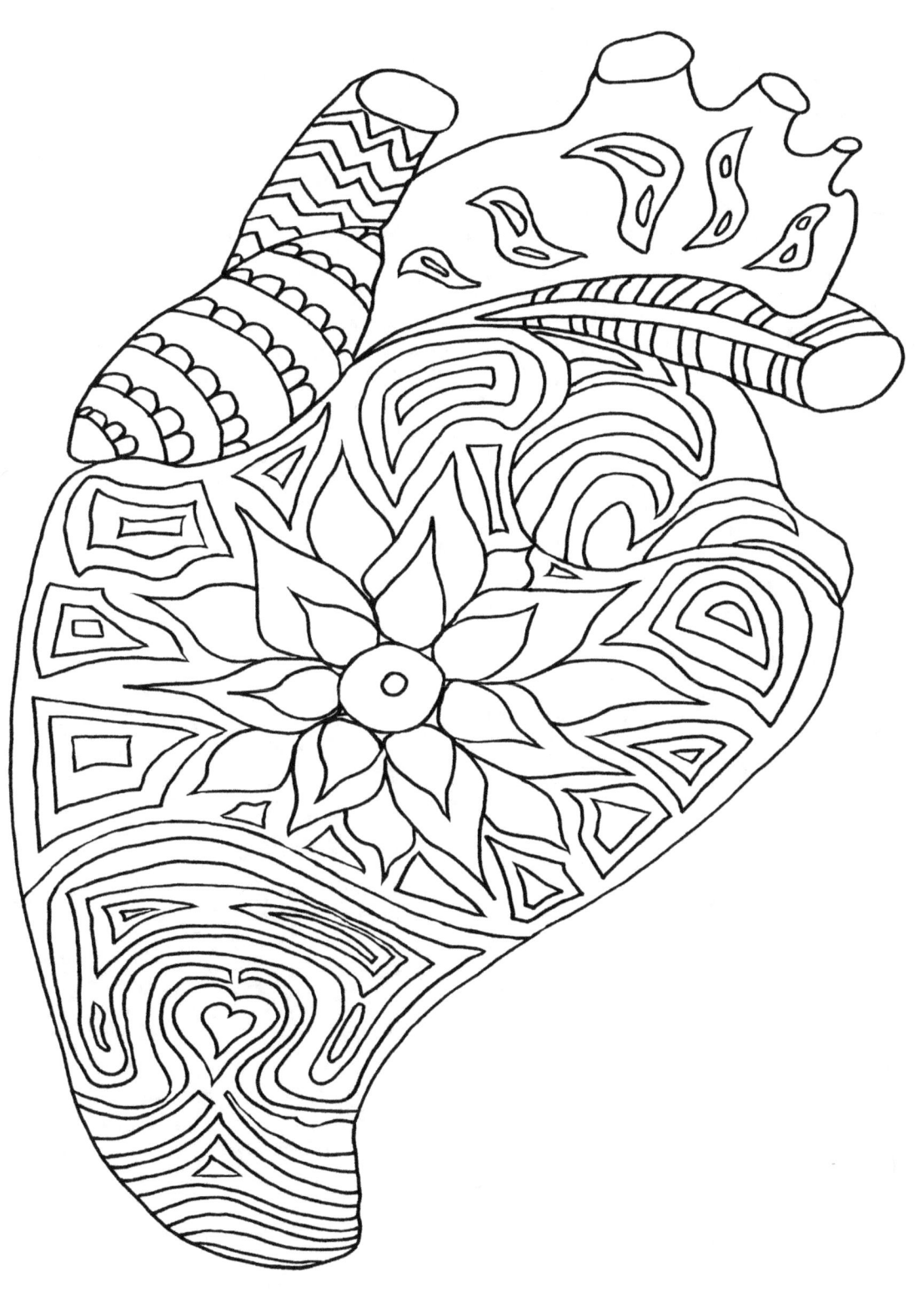

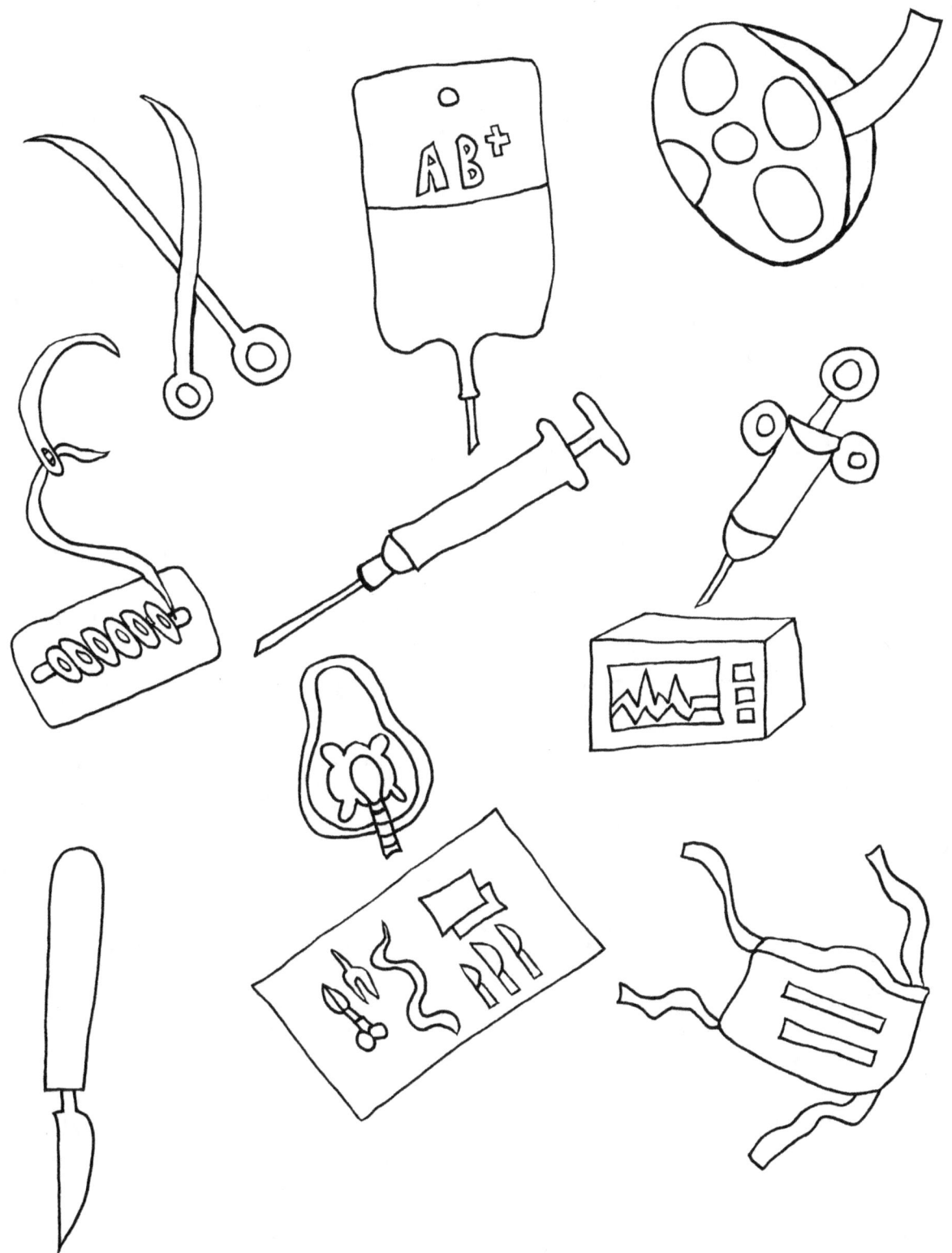

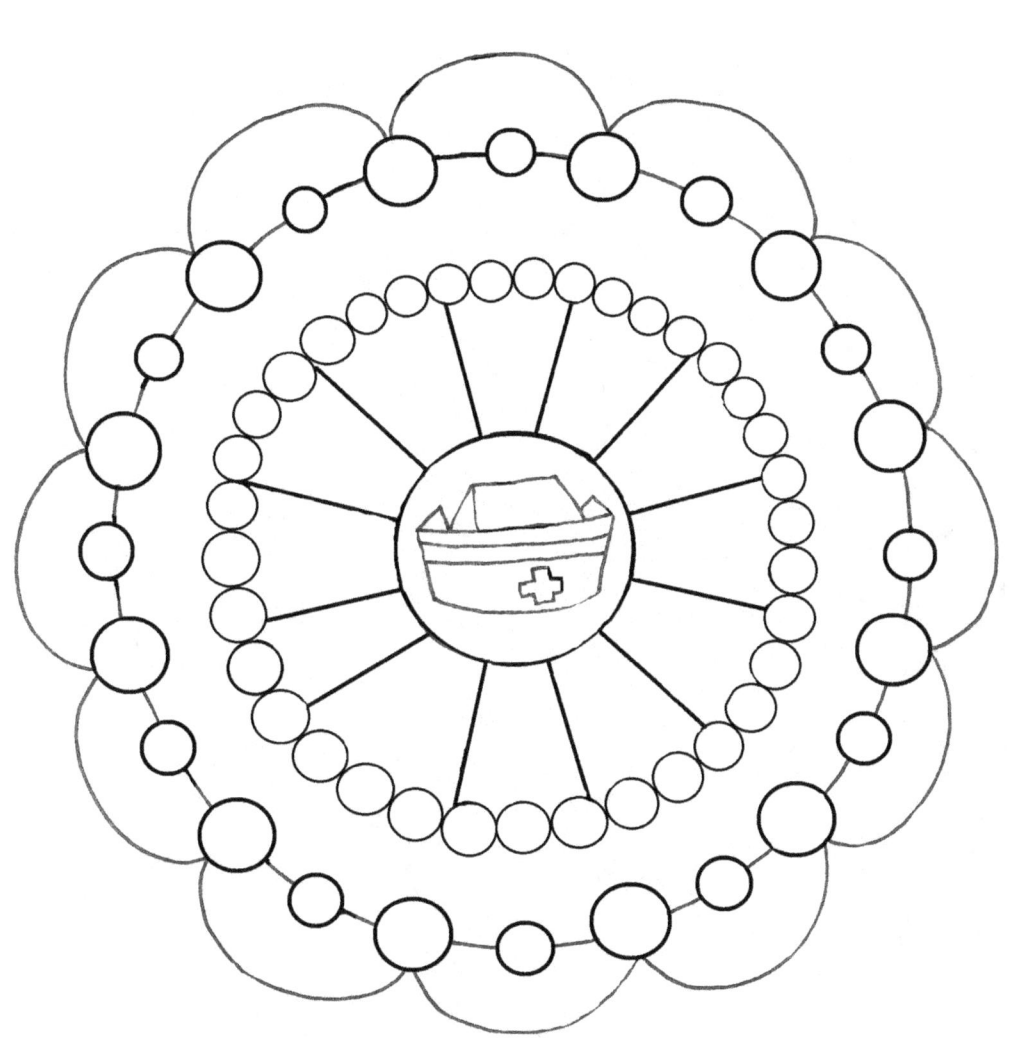

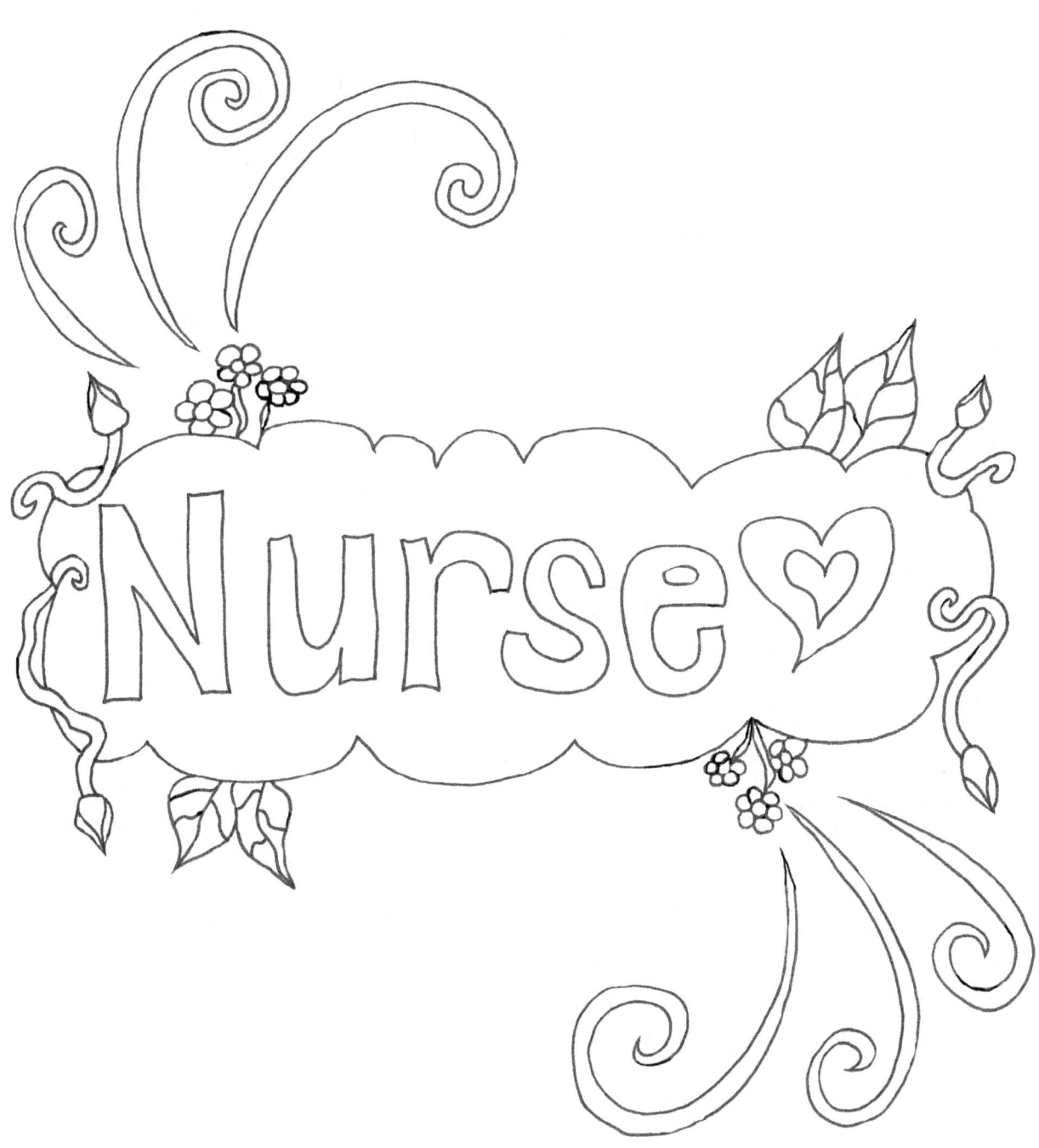

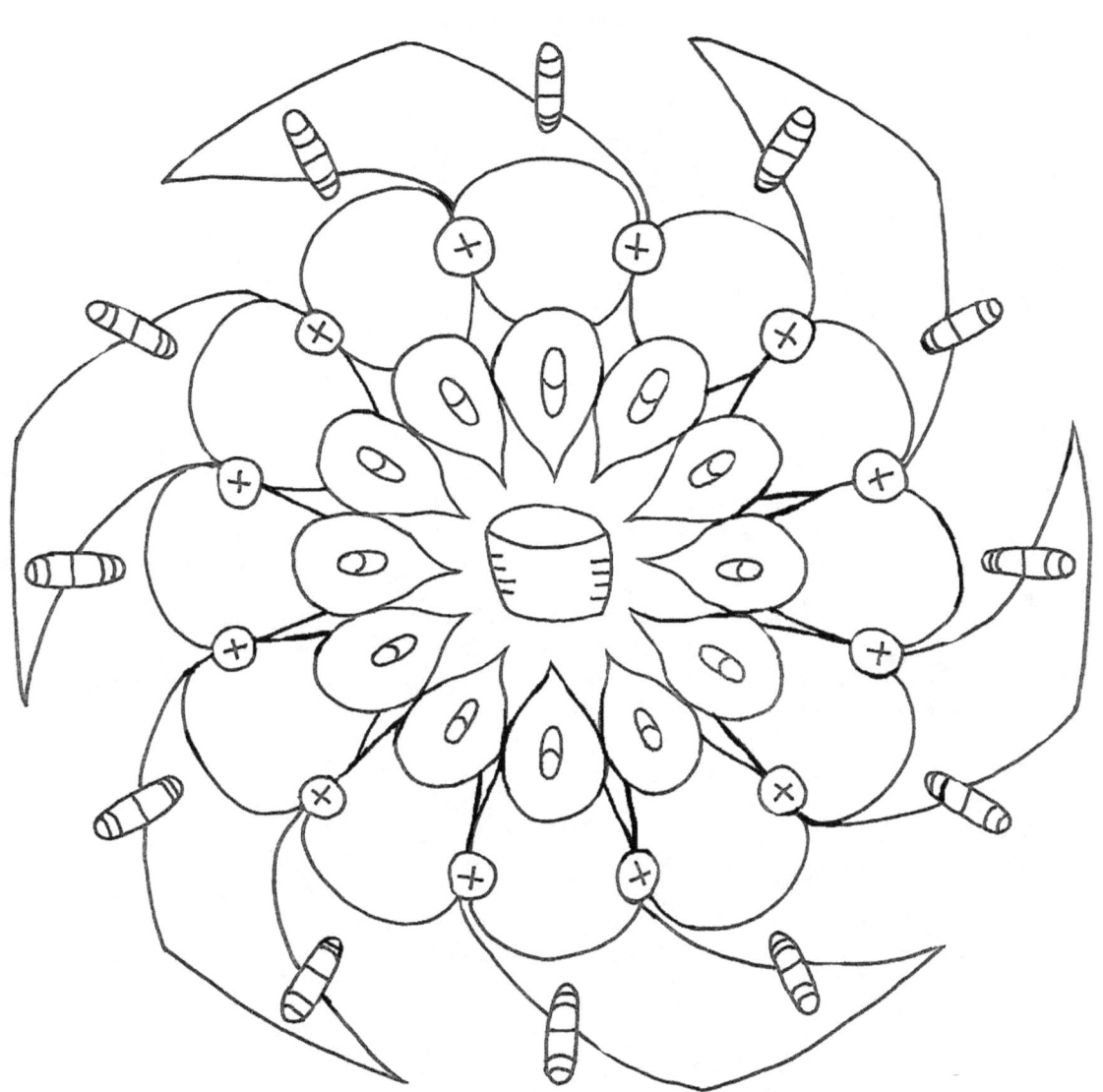

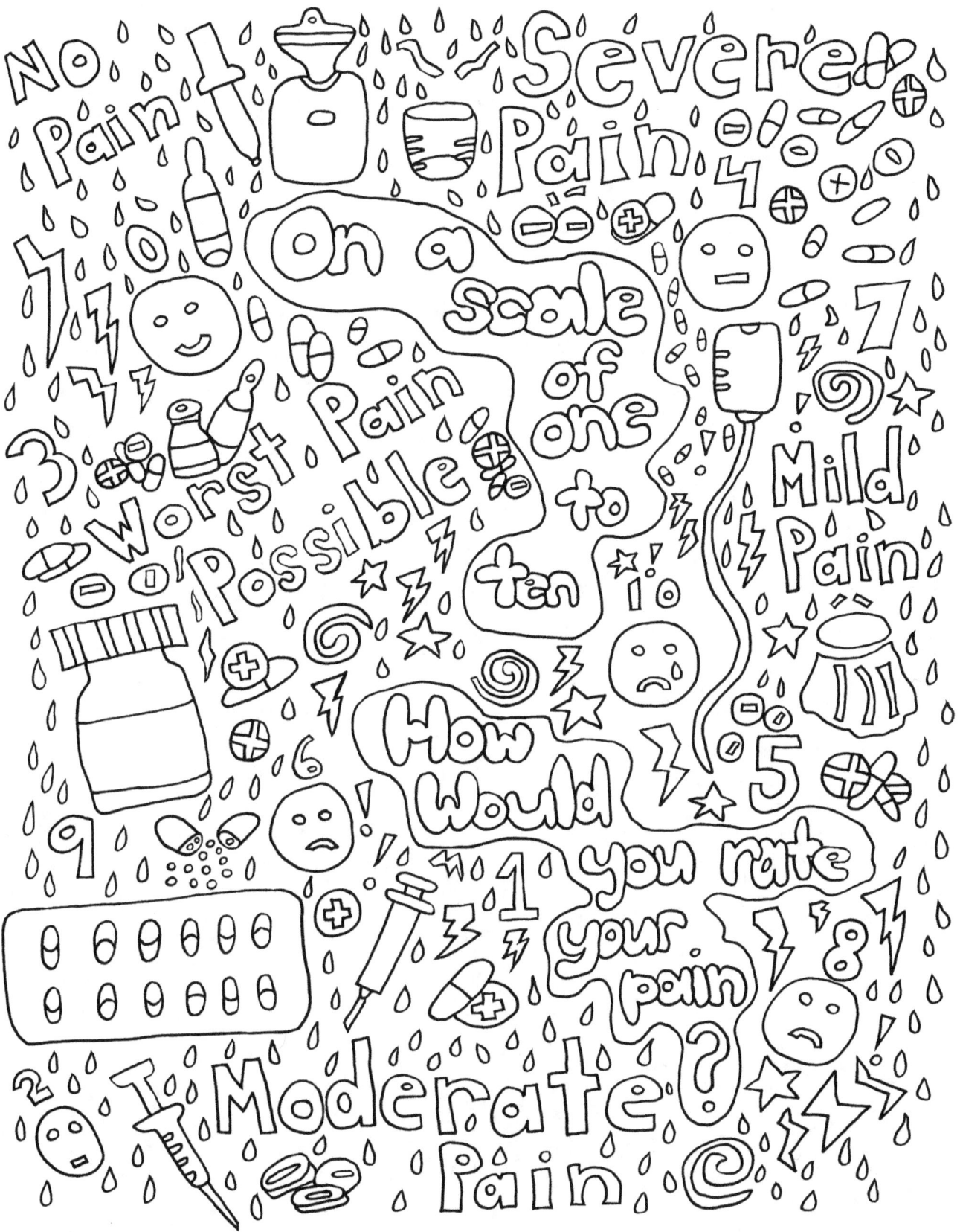

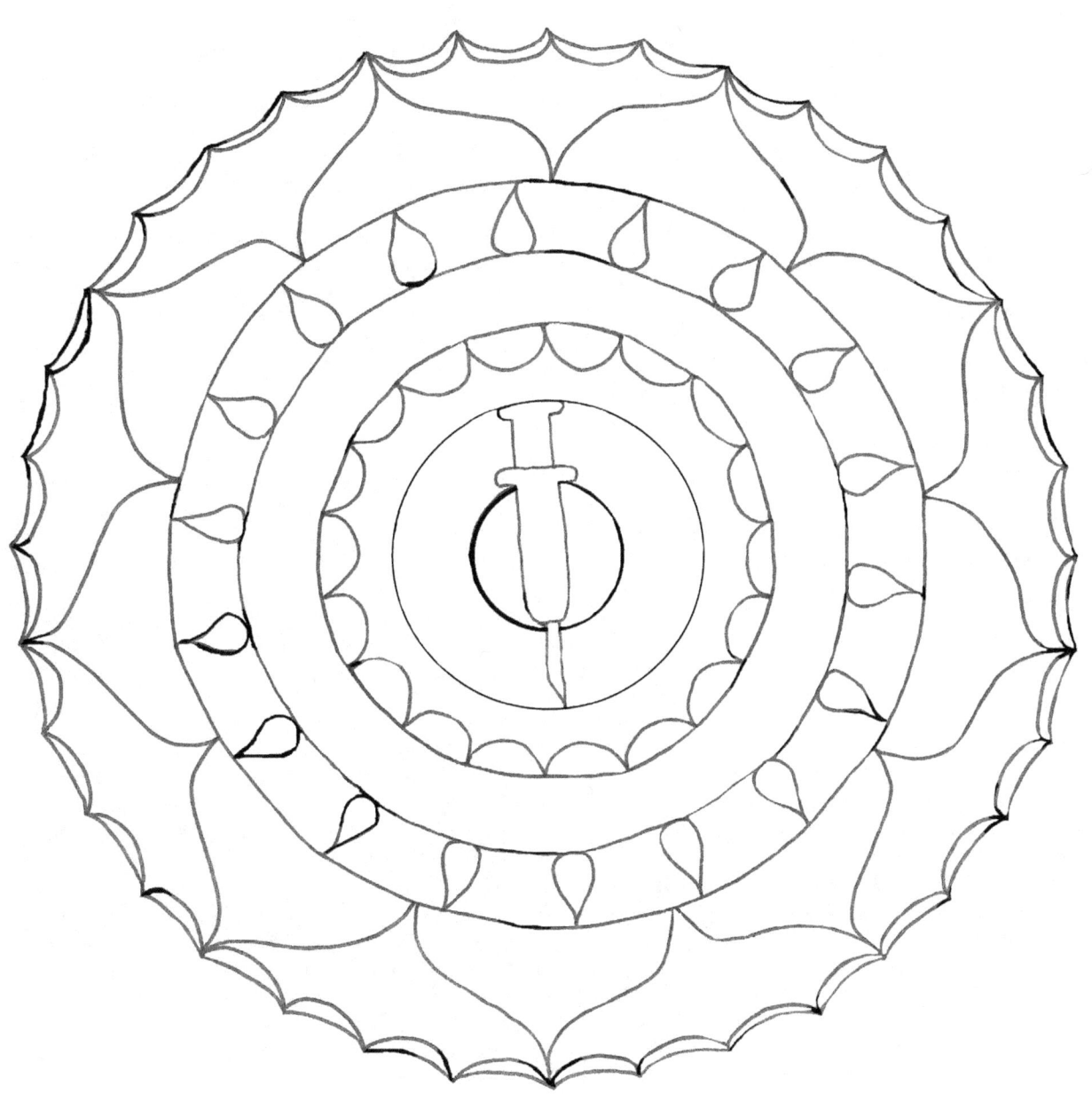

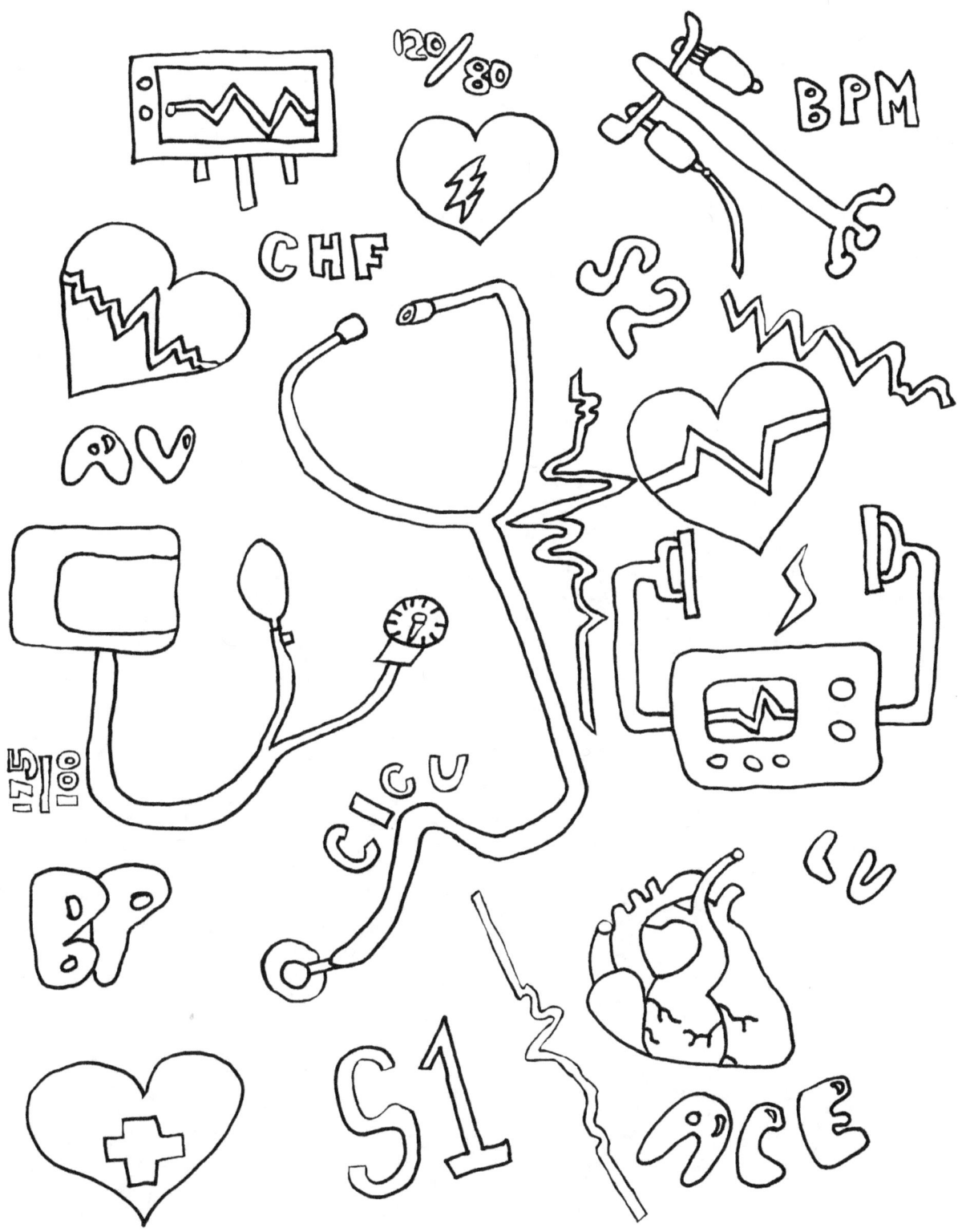

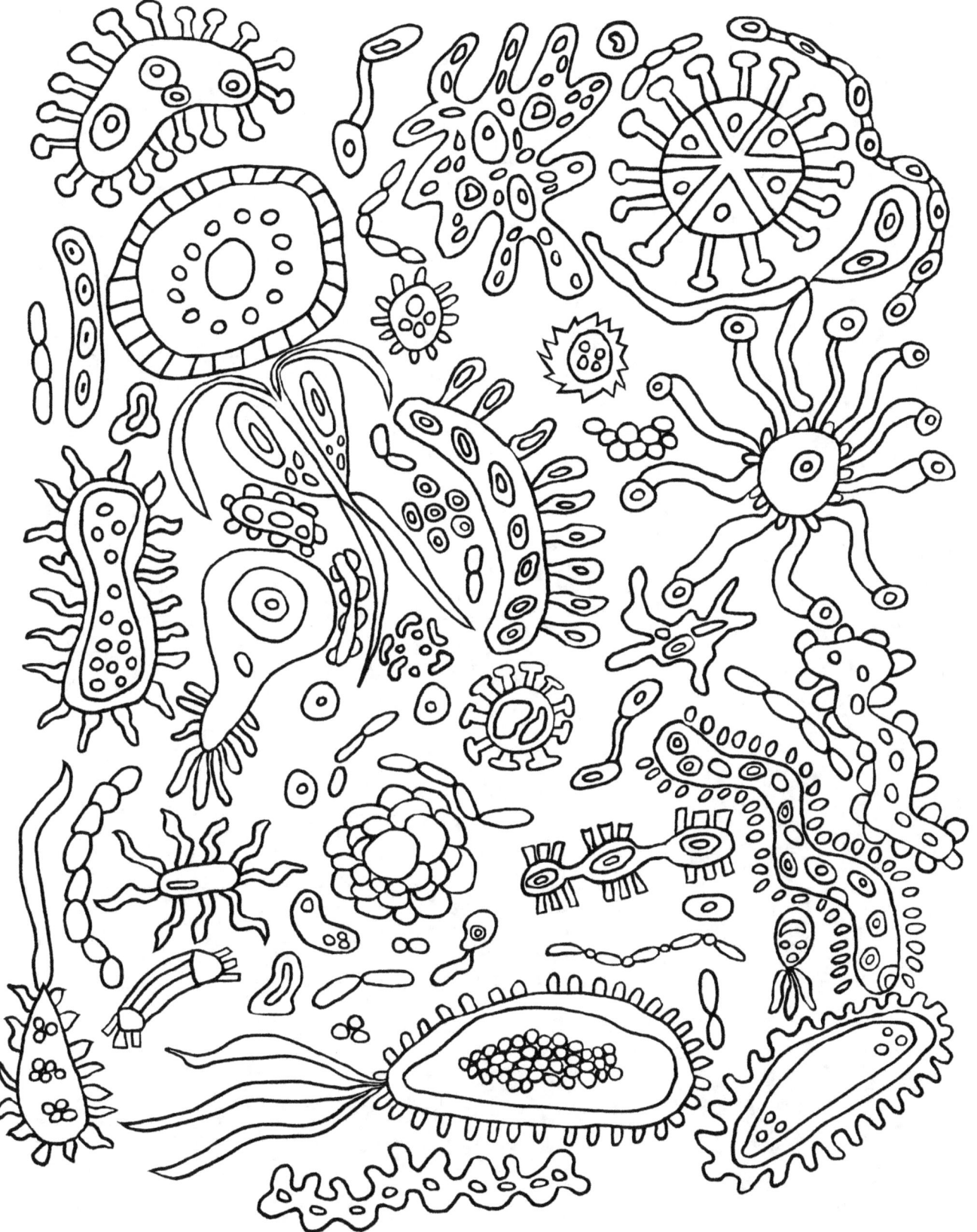

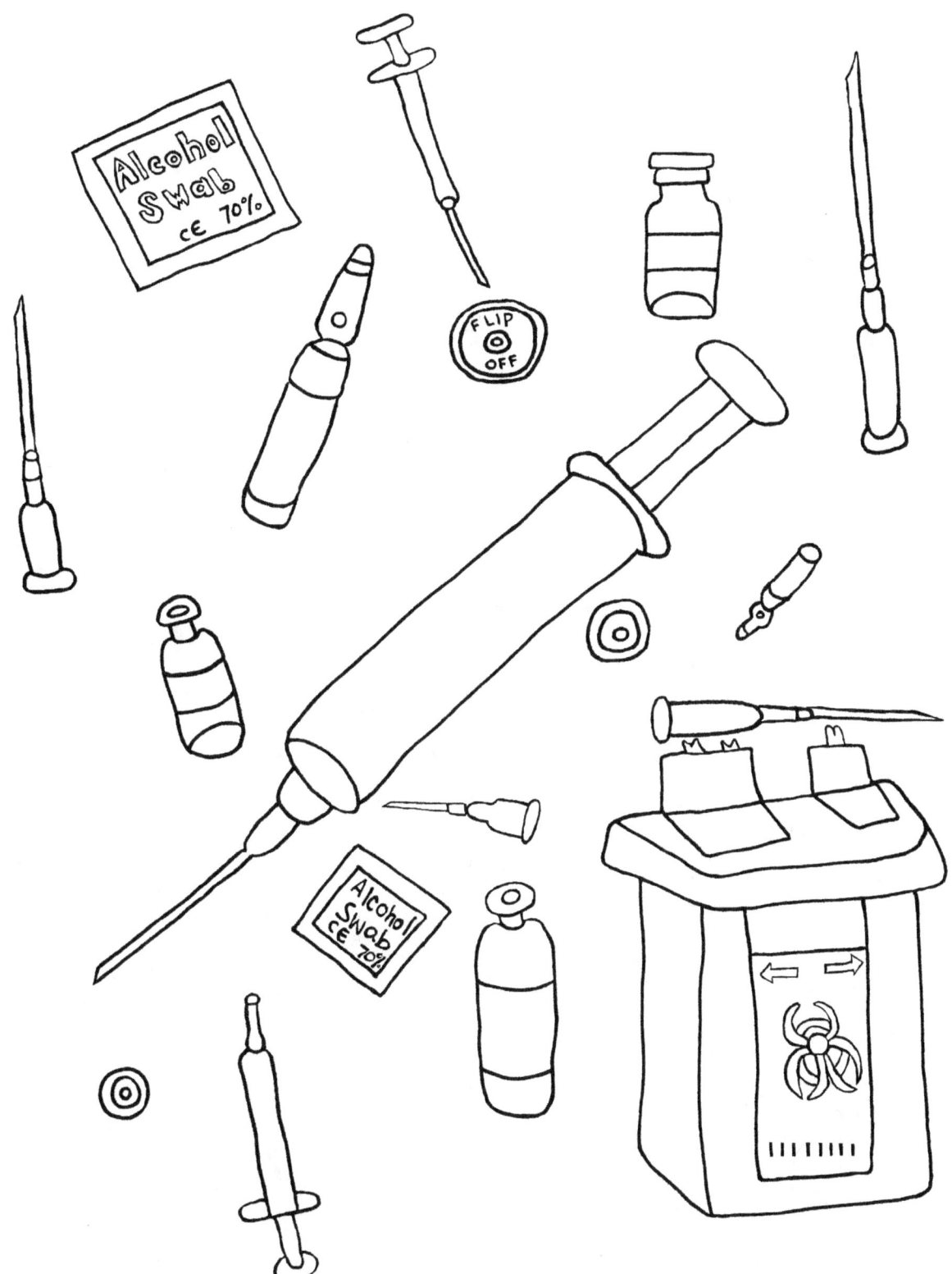

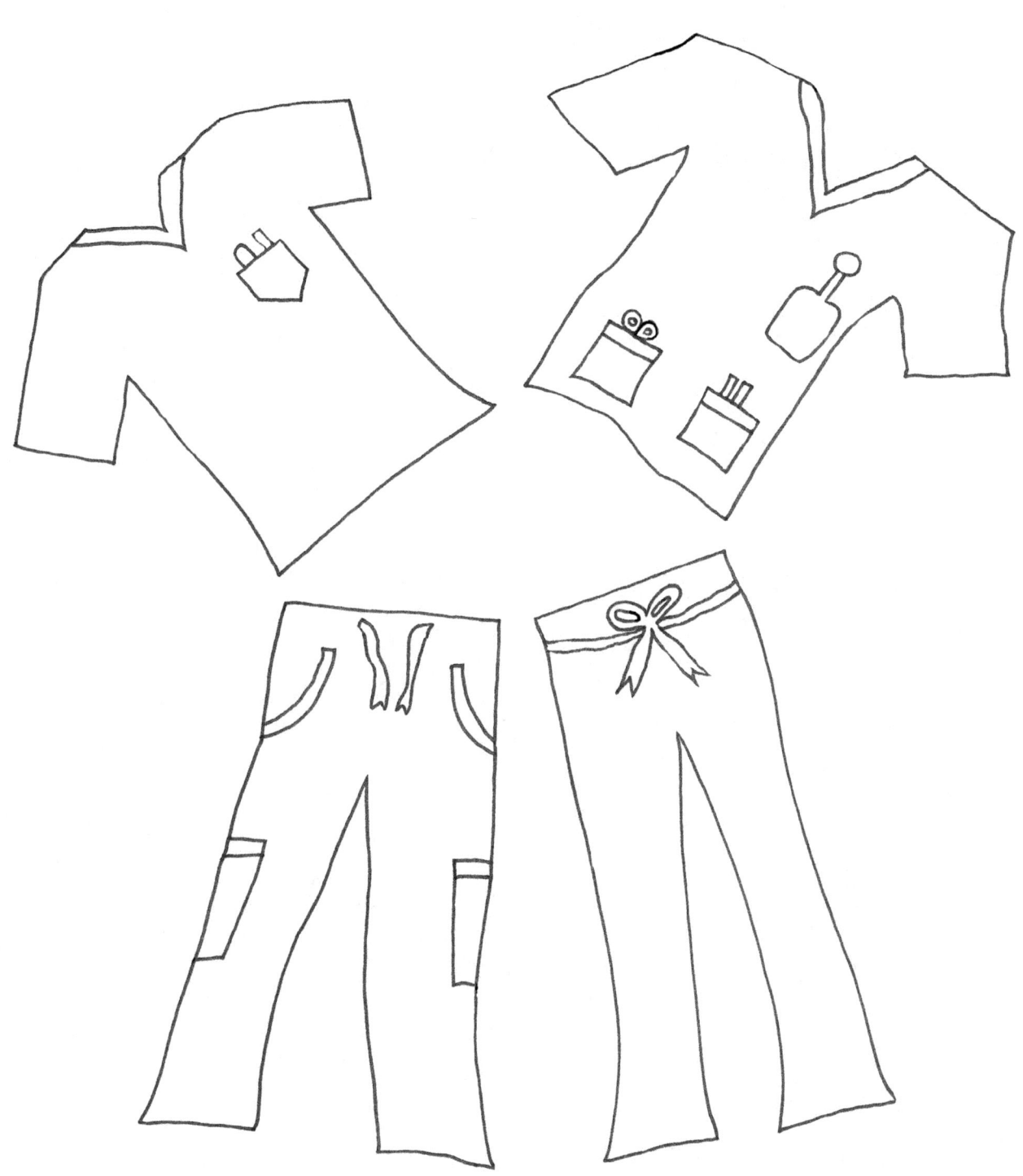

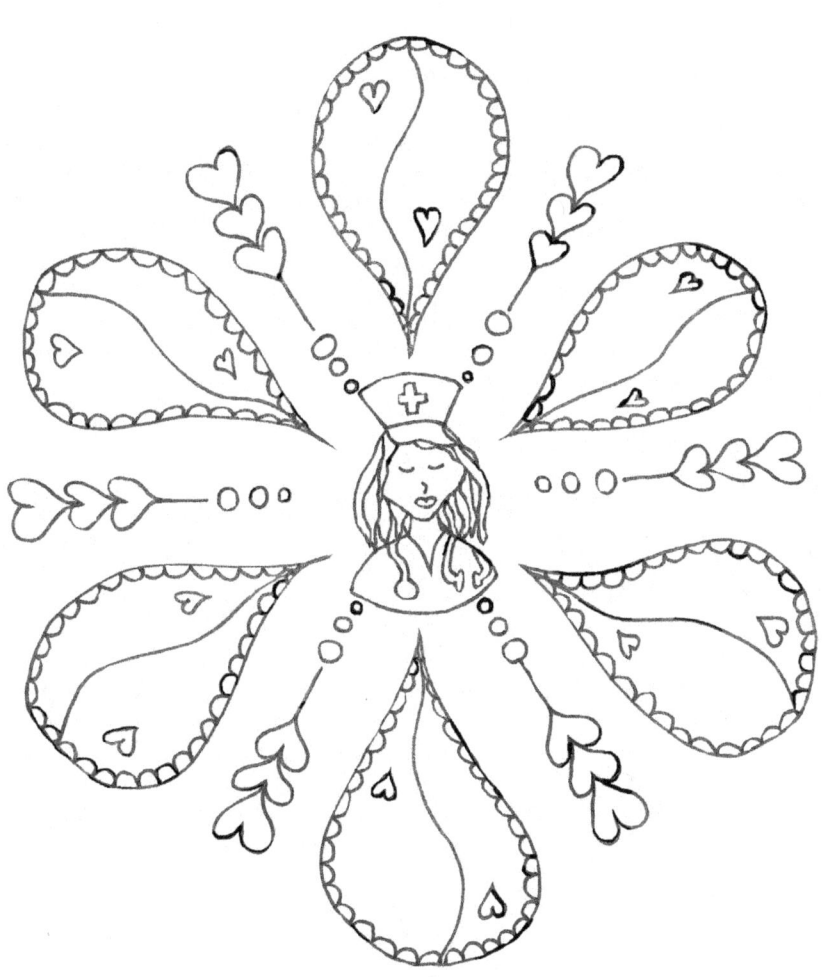

www.ingramcontent.com/pod-product-compliance
Lightning Source LLC
Chambersburg PA
CBHW062228220526
45471CB00009B/3397